VOLUME 1

Dick Loss Prevention

Make sure your dick doesn't fall off before
you die drunk and alone

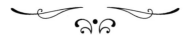

by Ryan Levis

◆ FriesenPress

Suite 300 - 990 Fort St
Victoria, BC, Canada, V8V 3K2
www.friesenpress.com

Copyright © 2015 by Ryan Levis
First Edition — 2015

Illustrations by Tyler Clarke and Nellie Hawthorn

ISBN
978-1-4602-6175-0 (Hardcover)
978-1-4602-6176-7 (Paperback)
978-1-4602-6177-4 (eBook)

1. Self-Help, Personal Growth, Sexuality

Distributed to the trade by The Ingram Book Company

Table of Contents

Acknowledgement
To all my supporters and loves-past, to
whom I am profoundly ingratiated.

The Classical Apology

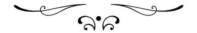

The wisdom within this book comes from my own mistakes. This knowledge came from an urgent need to change or die drunk and alone. I am no paragon of health, my recovery from anger and injury is, to this day, incomplete. However, with two long term injuries and a litany of fucked-up stories, through the haze of substance abuse I made it into treatment—unlike too many men.

When I began treatment for my physical and mental health (stemming from a vehicle-related head injury) improvement at eighteen was negligible. It took a savage break-up to pitch me into a full blown pattern of binge drinking. But it was only after I gave myself a crippling nail wound did I start to experience rapid decline. Damning regret and daily pain are the lasting impacts of my behavior between the ages of eighteen and twenty-two. Denial and shitty communication skills made it much worse. I was ambitious too. So basically I was a desperately loud-mouthed idiot; I found cannabis useful to curb my restlessness. But I was still drinking and screwing up relationships. My ego and cockiness left me isolated, entitled, and unhappy. I continued to produce comedy and Shakespeare. I got even bigger headed. Then I fucking won a national business title on the premise of a co-operative community housing model. All my bullshit-theatrics finally caught up to me and I collapsed. I couldn't make co-operative housing happen over-night it was literally going to take forever.

After reconciling that with myself over some time, I became a dedicated community healthcare researcher. Since then I've had some incredible training from the BC Schizophrenia Society, Vancouver Crisis Centre, Outpatient Mental Health & Addiction, and the local Men's Trauma Centre. I started seeing male behavioral protocols as major barriers to my happiness, my participation, and my relationships. So I started to schedule corny community activities for my lonely-ass self and just began showing up. It's tough to make change when we feel unworthy of compassion. Quaint self-care may seem odd for a man, but it is super relaxing and genuine fun.

Though I sincerely appreciate feedback, this book is a healthcare satire for dudes, the vernacular is intentional. I apologize in advance for my insensitive, derogatory language and flagrant displays of unpleasant themes.

If you don't like it, just make sure your dick doesn't fall off before you die drunk and alone.

Glossary of Terms

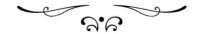

Amateurism – Voluntary participation in sports, activities, or trade with little or no experience and training. Avoid injuries, enter cautiously, and then commit. Participation will lead to meeting new people, which might include women!

Ants and Crusty Tissues – Indicators of repulsive domestic filth. There are few people who will be comfortable with men in this setting.

Apparently in Love – When abuse is present within a relationship where love once existed. Love is not love when there is violence, equity problems, yelling, or manipulative behaviour.

Ask for a Kiss – Mandatory first base consent. Asking to hold hands is advisable. The concept of consent scales up: ask for a kiss, ask to fondle her tits, ask to unbutton her pants, ask to lick her pussy, and ask to fuck her.

Backscratcher – A man without female sexual prospects. He is not homosexual; however, his only sexual options are men. He engages in gay sex without accepting his sexuality and is potentially volatile due to fear of exposure.

Barebacking – Sex without condoms. It can lead to pregnancy and spreading infections simultaneously. Condoms may be virtually free and by using them you command your genetic evolution more strategically.

Bargaining – When a man is negotiating for the return of an expired relationship, he's liable to vacillate between anger and depression. Use caution when bargaining, it is the opposite of acceptance and very likely to fail.

Beer Curls – When you are double fisting domestic beer in a style similar to bicep curls. The difference being one is a red flag for boozing and the other is a dedication to toned muscles.

Being Seen – Accepting and being vulnerable before the judgment of others. This includes, but is not limited to, exposing your flaws, past mistakes, dreams, desires, and fetishes. It might be embarrassing but it gets easier with time and communication. Facing the fear of weakness can provide a wealth of confidence and self-esteem.

Best Strokes – What a man is good at. Men are wise to play their strengths, and alleviate their weaknesses with effort and acknowledgement. To understand talents, men must also recognize flaws.

Cat Calling – Sexual harassment in the streets. Women will continue to evolve. The men who stay engaged in obsessive sexual objectification will not succeed sexually.

Compounding Problems – When a bad situation gets worse because of reactive behaviour. Don't do this. When shit gets bad, chill the fuck out and think about it. This is like binge drinking after a divorce and driving across town to beg your ex to come back. There are many ways to fuck shit up worse than it already is.

Conscientious Objector – One who intentionally rejects a cultural expectation. This can have a number of social impacts ranging from vilification to heroism.

Couch Diddlers – One who fondles his flaccid dick while sitting on the couch consuming entertainment and low quality food. He is unattractive due to his lack of ambition and pornography dependence. Likely, he also suffers numerous health and hygiene problems, which will go unaddressed until a health crisis.

C-U-Next-Tuesday – A clever disguise to say cunt.

Dick Brain – The relationship between the penis and the mind. It is most obvious when a man is rolling a condom down his shaft. The relationship between dick and brain ebbs and flows: a man should never be 100% brain or 100% dick.

Dick Impulse – A sexual urge that occurs in men potentially several times a day. It is an indicator of man's biological purpose and acts as a major motivator. Testosterone and sexual virility can be channeled into positive expression and need not always be flagrantly sexual. Community health depends on positive participation of men, not just their ejaculations.

Dick Philosophy – The values men associate with their penis. They exist and are highly personal. Men have a relationship with their dicks, their erections, and the orifices they hope to visit. Answer these questions: how to fuck, why to fuck, who to fuck, what to fuck, when to fuck before fucking up fucking. This involves understanding how to respond to rejection and commitment.

Douche Maneuver – When a guy tries to symbolically wash himself clean of any wrong-doing. He avoids punishment by out-doing his opponent with defensive wordplay. By repositioning blame on someone else, he identifies himself an idiot who won't take responsibility for how he affects people. This emotional avoidance is fundamentally manipulative and is an attempt to preserve that man's self-image at the expense of another.

Emotional Hangover – The result of a massive emotional shock. Though it might imply boozing, alcohol is not necessary. However, it does require a significant conflict. A divorce, a death, or a massive failure can result in a lingering period of misery. How you handle yourself during this period sets the trajectory for your recovery.

Enamel – The stuff your teeth are covered with. Enamel ranks a five on Mohs Hardness Scale (whatever the fuck that means). Basically, teeth aren't hard—just average. The expense of dentures is extensive and on top of that, dentures are fucking terrible.

Exit Before You Escalate – Recognizing the physical symptoms of masculine emotional duress and relieve aggression before it becomes violence. Some rage indicators include: blood pressure spikes, redness in the face, stammering, hitting inanimate objects, or yelling. If you notice any of these symptoms, exit the conflict immediately.

Change – A long-standing philosophical conversation about the nature of personal change. This book is for men whom (fancy-pants) psychologists might consider "pre-contemplators." Swooshy academia on this subject exists in far more thorough (but boring) contexts. There is a plethora of pre-existing institutional and community efforts that seek to foster healthy change.

F.I.N.E. – An acronym for "Fucked up, Insecure, Neurotic, and Explosive." These feelings are virtually invisible until a trigger or a crisis occurs. It is easy to hide behind barriers of emotional deflection but it will not serve long-term relationships and results in lashing out.

Facts – Not facts. Question everything. This book presents masculine dilemmas with often no clear path. Men will encounter situations in which all of their (perceived) choices are bad. Alternative choices may exist but may not fit into the code of masculinity. For example: if a therapist is available for a man, but that man is too ashamed to seek help, help is not available. Fact, not a fact.

Female Ideal of Masculinity – How the desires of women shape the behaviours of men. Unfortunately, however, if men reach this invisible bar (Prince Charming), they will quickly discover that they haven't. This is men's susceptibility to being a tool on a singular sexual journey. It invalidates his more complex emotions. To be a positive male in their community (who women like), the good men pick and choose the components of culture that work for them and avoid the intangible perfection seen in romance movies.

Food Documentaries – Movies about the human food chain. In North America we are the majority consumers and yet the minority population. Globalization provides us with a significant challenge for the next generations. These films will give men some perspective and appreciation for the global challenges ahead of us as a species—in turn, that will make men well-rounded.

Go Fuck Yourself – A literal insult. It means masturbation is his only option to be sexually satisfied and that he has no sexual partners. It is a great insult.

Fucked Up Life Before 30 – A depressed state of mind. Many young people have been carrying this psychological disposition. Our economic recession, rising student debt, wealth disparity, technological-emotional disharmony, and the prevalence of global war reporting have augmented this feeling of youth gloom. It begets helplessness, stress, and future sickness. It gets worse when student debt protests eventually evolve into housing riots.

Fuckup – When a man's behaviour results in punishment known to the community or someone close to him. Isolated fuckups don't count, they just makes him a closet fuckup. Obviously, avoid fuckups. Not so obviously, however, also be prepared to accept terms of restitution and the consequences: learn from fuckups.

Gape Response – When a man's first response upon seeing a woman is to eye-fuck her tits and ass. Individuals who gape at women are uncomfortable around them and jealous around sexually successful men. Through bystander intervention and speaking out against objectification of women, we can curb this isolating behaviour. These men are creepy and lonely.

Grannies with Butt Plugs – Sex at extremes. It is possible to have a high sex drive in your senior years. The women engaging in this type of pornography are doing it for money. To have that kind of sex life in your later years, try getting your shit together today.

Hangover Depression – Misery following a period of binge drinking. Poisoning oneself can provide momentary enjoyment; however, factors such as dehydration, fucking up, and an irregular diet will decrease a man's ability to be happy and productive. Don't expect him to be vigorous or enthusiastic while ignoring his alcohol addiction and emotional problems.

Hosting Friends and Lovers – Healthy well-adjusted behaviour. Making plans to have company requires a reasonable degree of hygiene, the ability to socialize with others, and the capability of future planning. All of these are necessary skills for a sustainable relationship. Most begin as a guest and transition into being a host. Being a good guest is good practice.

Hyper-Localized Growing – Personally growing food-bearing plants. Very sexy, and it never goes out of style.

In-Bed Sex – Having intercourse in the place where you sleep. Your room is presumably the sexiest place in your home. Lovers should be comfortable there and the sheets should be free of crumbs, stinks, and stains. Your bedroom is your sexual sanctuary.

Indentured Housewives – A condition referring to how religion and government can (and do) control the reproductive rights of women. The rapid social evolution of women has made this concept impossible for men to enforce domestically. Today, a man who seeks an indentured housewife should find one predisposed to that kind of work rather than operate on out-dated expectations of female-domestic slavery.

Insecure Intelligencia – Intelligent and powerful men who have poor conflict skills and are culturally isolated. They are easily intimidated, chronically terrified (by economics or health), and give back to the community with a 'white savior complex' more fervent than that of young aid workers in

Africa. Power combined with fear results in retaliatory behaviour when challenged, and these rich folks are prone to ignorance, apathy, and overkill.

Integrity of Intention – Speaking clearly about intention and ambitions (sexually and professionally). This includes asking a woman on a date, but also includes being honest about your goals in general.

Internet Dopes – Men who stay up late to masturbate and write asshole comments online. Yuck. Any comment posted after 1 a.m. is highly suspicious. They lack sexual access and are bitter because of it.

Jack Yourself – Different from masturbation in that it includes a self-aggrandizing aspect. Imaginary sexual scenarios artificially conflate a person's ego and impose vain sexual dominance.

John – A man who rents a prostitute. There is no love for these transactions in the community. They are the ones who will be punished for any foul play. These men are well advised to be emotionally stable. Never redirect internal anger onto the prostitute.

Libido – The urge to fuck. This is different from sexual magnetism in that one can have a large libido but attract no sexual partners. Essentially, it does not require skill or practice. Libido is simply the strength of one's sexual drive. It can be problematic when a man is rejected frequently. Such a man should diversify his strategy because he is likely operating on out-dated male behavioral protocols.

Lusty Homo-Social Sex Talk – When guys in groups talk about how they'd fuck a specific person. When men sit around discussing how they'd fuck someone if they could, it shows how the whole group has grown into sexless trolls. As one man explains his sexual vision, he simultaneously sexually stimulates his male peers to engage in sexual thinking. These guys have been checking out babes together for decades. In the process, they have gotten accustomed to having little erections around each other. It should not be a surprise when one straight guy sucks off another straight guy: they're obsessed with sex but can't get any. See 'backscratcher'.

Man-Camp – When dudes go camping. It's great! Highly advisable. Don't drink and drive (or shoot guns, or go boating, or mountaineering). Guys do a ton of awesome shit together. Sure, it gets unhinged. Sure, a safety meeting often isn't that focused on safety. So long as they don't hurt themselves, they should have fun and go fucking wild—safely.

Man-Maneuver – When a guy justifies stupid behaviour based on being a man. It is a sign of his ignorance of male-privilege.

Masculine Infallibility Complex – The idea that men must be the protector. The problem here is that every man is guaranteed to fail. When he punishes himself because of weakness he reinforces his flaws with anger. This doesn't serve anyone.

Masturbation Station – An at-home shrine dedicated to the consumption of pornography. For the sake of future sex, try to make it less obvious. Keep it tidy and dispose of the tissues before they get crusty.

Masturbatory Death Grip – The extraordinary strength that our dominant hand can apply when it strokes our cock. This self-applied force is unrealistic compared to a real vagina. Use only two or three fingers when you whack off to avoid desensitizing your dick from what is naturally less tight.

Medean Crisis – When women retaliate against men in response to male negligence. This is like a football team being poisoned after a known sexual assault is thrown out of the court. If justice continues to fail women regarding issues of extreme male ignorance, they are fully capable of taking control of the situation by their own means.

Men Become Suicidal After Divorce – Based on the stereotype of men being pre-conditioned as solely emotionally dependant on women makes it no surprise that men might overreact during divorce. Men who respond to female abandonment with violence have been foolishly trained to expect woman to take care of all their needs.

Mental Blocks – When we ignore a persistent issue even though having the solution would relieve us immensely. This could be taking out the garbage, eating well, stopping smoking, or getting fit. We can ignore problems for a variety of reasons. These are all mental blocks. Try to identify these hang-ups and fix them. Clean up your mind a bit, but don't expect love to automatically come flooding in.

Mental Health Gauntlet – A long process of acknowledging, accommodating, and growing beyond old hang-ups. This is a worthwhile but uncomfortable process. It requires a man to see that he's been fucked up for a long time and that it is okay to recover from that.

Muffin-Top (aka: Love Handle, Amateur in Spandex) – The bulge of fat that pokes out over your belt-line when your pants are too tight.

Naked People March – A public event for naked people as some type of social-political stunt—possibly art. Don't necessarily become a nudist but recognize that these events are specifically designed to help everyone love their body. Just show up to watch a Naked Bike Ride or a Pride Parade.

Natural Smell – The fragrance of a man's home and body without artificial perfumes. Ideally a man's smell doesn't repulse his company. Cleaning, hygiene, and not letting shit mould behind the refrigerator will help to fix this.

Negative Learning Environment – How, where, and when we have learned our shitty habits. Bad behaviour is reinforced by group thought. This is how dudes have learned that binge drinking and vomiting is a rite of passage into college masculinity.

Negativity Bias – How our ego is more attracted to negative events in our life than positive. For example, if by some miracle you are out on a date and everything is going well but at some point your baldness is criticized, you are sure-as-shit gonna remember that criticism more than the nice stuff.

Regular Emotions – The range of feelings between happiness and anger. There are thousands of emotions and they often exist simultaneously. Certain circumstances draw out big emotional responses. Because men lack emotional identification skills, they suffer by reacting impulsively rather than responding thoughtfully. The differentiation lies in a man's ability to identify his complex regular emotions.

Past Expectations – The lessons learned that we are convinced will become a repeat pattern. This ranges from how we behave around women to the outcomes of exercise.

Pattern-Jackass – When men keep fucking up despite obvious red flags. Ignoring problems is the root of why men fuck up so much. These patterns are hard to break because they are likely rooted in early childhood development, trauma, and out-dated masculine protocols that restrict his (perceived) ability to make positive change.

Poop Log – A chart that tracks bowel movements. The best way
to curb uncomfortable shitting is to be mindful of the quality of
shit and the impact that diet may have had on that shit.

Population Crisis – Explained better by professionals in global health. However,
if men continue in this pattern of health-neglect they will self-sterilize. Men are
facilitating their own genetic decline by not taking their healthcare seriously.

Pornophile – One who loves pornography more than real human
physical contact. This has likely occurred through decades of
sexual and social isolation. It is the formation of a false belief
that human love has passed by or we are unworthy.

Pride Barrier – Inhibits men from participating in fun due to a
flawed masculine behavioural protocol that rejects basic kindness for fear of becoming emasculated by the group.

Proctologist – A doctor who specializes in issues pertain-
ing to the anus, rectum, prostate, and colon.

Rapey – A man's behaviour that is deemed as creepy or sexually unwel-
come by an often female second party. It can be defined by a man creating
emotional or sexual expectations that are unknown to that second party.

Rebound Perversions – When a man acts like sport-fucking post-divorce (or
abandonment) will somehow satisfy his feelings of rejection and loneliness.

Recovery Errors – The mistakes, relapses, and false confidences a man
carries when he is attempting to make personal change. When trying to
self-improve, it is normal to fuck-up a little. Don't start all over again angry
and disappointed. Try again next time from the same point of progress.

Relationship Equity – The aspect of a relationship that makes both
parties equally powerful and deserving of respect and support.

Relationship Loss – Rejection, abandonment, and grief. How
men respond to relationship loss is more important than the loss
itself. There are many ways to suck at life; sometimes unimproved
flaws become extremely divorceable. A man ought to seek self-
improvement rather than punish those who have rejected him.

Re-Toxify – Treating a hangover with more alcohol or another substance. Though it might work momentarily, it is a sure-fire path to dependency.

Self-Advocacy – Accepting that we are worthy of support, kindness, and encouragement despite ourselves. This is when a man sticks up for himself while seeking to get his needs met.

Sexualized – The pattern of appreciating a woman's beauty, not for its own sake but for a desire to fuck her as well. It serves only to intimidate women, paint the man as a douche bag, and ostracize him from romantic love.

Sexually Successful – The act of having two children and raising them with healthy fatherly values and their success in mind.

Shakes – A symptom of withdrawal, serious illness, or severe emotional agitation. This is an imminent health crisis.

Shit-Mouth – When men talk about themselves like they are the king-shit. Bravado, arrogance, hostility, and lies are all symptoms of having shit-mouth.

Shlubby Existence – How we live when we are in denial of our long-term health needs; a man with poor hygiene, social skills, and dietary habits. He suffers from lethargy, apathy, bitterness, and emotional numbness/dependency. His future health concerns are extraordinary.

Sissy Bitch – An insult of emasculation. It infers that an individual is both a homosexual and a woman. The insult is tragically unoriginal and poorly thought out. It suggests that being a woman or a homosexual is globally bad. This is not true. The user of this insult restricts his social circle to douche bag men and increases his likelihood of becoming a backscratcher.

Social Magnetism – The ability of a person to attract attention from nearby humans. The localized response can be positive or negative.

Sport Fucking – The practice of fucking to relieve emotional incapacity and keep score between douche bags. It is conducted by millions of men as a method to prove their masculinity to their male peers. It is essentially a queer homo-social ranking system by which dudes evaluate other dudes' dicks and their ability to have sex.

Spousal Supervision – A wife or girlfriend overseeing a man's behaviour so that his stupidity doesn't hurt himself, others, and his children.

Squat – A position to better evacuate your bowels. There are special squat stations available to modify the western toilet to accommodate this more efficient style of shitting. Not recommended for the fat, weak, and inflexible—or injured.

Stroker Warmer – Like a gelatin heat pad that is shaped especially for your pocket-pussy so that when you begin your masturbation session, the artificial orifice is pre-heated.

Stupidity Honour – When men congratulate each other for undertaking unnecessary risks and surviving. Men re-enforce each other's stupidity this way and make an accidental death, rape allegation, or permanent injury all but guaranteed within their peer group.

Topy Soles – A protective sole to have applied by a cobbler that will prevent your nice shoes from wearing out too quickly. They can add years of use to fancy shoes.

Traditional Hours of Fucking – Typically considered the evening or after-dinner hours. However, divergence from this norm can prove invigorating to matured sexual relationships.

Uggo – Folks who are ugly on the outside and let that ugliness permeate their core.

Unlearned Fun – How we have learned to define adult fun. Weekends, videogames, binges, and sex are minor in the scope of how fun life can be. Men must re-learn how to have fun if they seek to make change.

Unquestioning Servitude – When men invest emotionally to only one person ever and become doormats to their partner out of their fear of loneliness. Sometimes more effort will not save a doomed relationship. A man in this state of mind risks rage or self-destructive behaviors upon divorce.

Vagina-Like (and Anus-Like) Tools – Also known as strokers or masturbation aids. They come in a variety of styles, shapes, colours, and tightness.

Welcome, Jackass

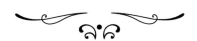

So you've got this book now, do ya? Great. Now, men, we can't change without first thinking about change. Wrong. Accidents happen and force change upon us. But really, whose job is it to change us, and who is going to define our success? That's right. You are gonna change you. You are gonna define what your successful change means. I'm just a wise old jackass who is slightly further along in the evolution of men. We're gonna go on a magic fucking journey, okay? I'm gonna present a number of stupid man-isms and accuse you of them all.

All men have fucked up somehow, so let's just call it what it is: misdirected manliness. As dudes, we are prone to behaving like assholes (or wieners) out of fear of facing our readily emasculated ineptitudes. Every man has serious character flaws. We hide our weaknesses to save-face among dudes, and by doing so we fuck our shit up even more. Let's pry ourselves from this delusional cell of numb masculinity and experience life without the self-destructive man-bullshit that sabotages our relationships and our satisfaction.

Don't get angry at me, boy. Mostly what I've done here is expose myself as a severely flawed jackass who is as guilty of stupidity as anyone. The difference, however, is that I'm trying to recover from this shit rather than just pretend that living like a fuckup is okay. Ideally, this is a prevention guide, so take notes, use highlighters, and maybe even make a mind-map of some stuff. However, if you are on par with me on a stupidity/time ratio, then we can classify this as a bro-couragement guide.

Prepare yourself for a battery of manly conflicts that scrutinizes your right to masculinity while offering tips for (unlikely) future relationships.

If this book causes self-piteous weeping or resentment towards owning the world's most callous self-help book, then consider seeking professional medical attention. Understand that no one has all these problems; most men are half-decent already.

I assume that no man wants to die drunk, alone, and emasculated. Who does? Having relationships will support a man's life-long development; however, he must start by supporting himself. Men who are pre-exposed to health problems (ie: illness and/or stupidity) will be less likely to sexually succeed. Over the next generations, if we factor in divorce rates and underemployment, we might discover that men will be taking care of their own health needs more. It behoves us, gentlemen, to sincerely consider an emotional future where we rely less heavily on women for our physical and mental health maintenance.

Socially and biologically, it is an unusual time. For the first time in written history, men have lost some sexual entitlement! It is not a surprise that men would be confused by this change. Gentlemen, we are experiencing the bafflingly rapid evolution of the species. A new set of masculine expectations has been added on to the already long list of male behavioural protocols. Simply put, that new expectation is that women are extremely capable.

To begin this journey, do not become defensive and say, "Fuck you, Ryan, I do respect women," just read-on. This book will show men how to accommodate, articulate, and participate in this evolutionary change of sexual expression. The behavioural conflicts presented in this book will help us understand ourselves and support our self-improvement. The point being, a man who can articulate his complex philosophy of personal growth will have more sex and better relationships.

This book presents behavioural conflicts for men to wrestle with internally. The hope is that by hosting these internal conflicts, men will be better prepared for conflicts in real life.

Book 1
The Basic Chapters

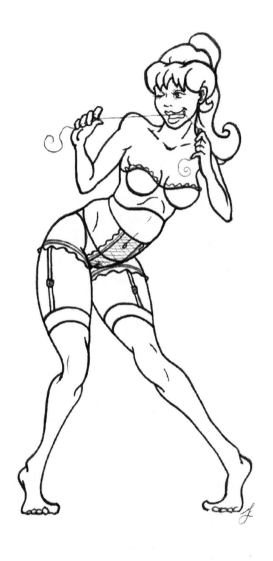

1.

Floss Your Fucking Teeth!

There is nothing less sexy than tooth decay. Nothing. If you want to commit your sex life to coal mines or data entry or call centres, then by all means let those pearly white teeth go brown. Lovers will not thrilled to introduce her family to a man with evident tooth decay. The current cost of everything is rising. A visit to the dentist will likely cost somewhere between $100 and $300. I bet the average budget (if average people made budgets) does not accommodate the cost of dentistry. Unfortunately then the maintenance of average teeth falls squarely onto our own self-discipline. Fuck.

Flossing is important, okay? I've seen a nineteen year old with tooth decay; he's gonna have a hard time getting a decent job. He's a broke-ass entertainer who doesn't even smile. So how the hell is he supposed to avoid dying drunk, unsuccessful, and alone? Answer: retroactive flossing (does not exist). If it has come to blackened teeth, a man has seriously miscalculated his long-term goals. I mean, really, the mild discomfort and expense of dental hygiene is much more attractive than the denial of tooth decay. We will get old. Gravity kills. Our teeth will get worse. By our eighteenth birthday we're past our prime but we probably stopped flossing at ten.

Not only does tooth decay make a man very unattractive, the effects are virtually irreversible. Dentures are not a good alternative to healthy teeth. If we're so misguided to ignore the dentist in our annual budget then we sure as shit are not planning the expense of false teeth. The cost of living is going up; pensioners have ostensibly hoarded all the money and "benefit plans" are mostly a goddamn myth. Stubborn old goats like Granddad had the benefit of an indentured housewife who forced him to visit a dentist. Nowadays we're screwed. It's on us. If a wife leaves our shabby asses toothless, so be it.

Men love eating meat. We ravage salty roasted nuts. Chewy candies are fucking fantastic! Lose those teeth and we lose our ability to enjoy eating stuff. Unfortunately, the underemployed (or un-nagged) male can't or won't afford dentistry, which sucks big time. We can blame the government or the economy or even blame genetics, but blame doesn't solve rotting teeth. What it really comes down to is this: floss your fucking teeth, every fucking day. Supposedly, we should see the dentist twice a year, but when expenses out-weigh revenues, seeing a dentist every half-decade is sadly more realistic. That means we have to take care of those babies by ourselves—no one will ever floss for us. A cavity or a root canal costs as much as rent. To make matters worse, if we fail address the problem, tooth loss can necessitate prostitution, and that's not cheap either.

Not only do teeth process food, they are used for talking too. Do you remember that kid with a speech impediment that was mocked? If we lose our teeth, we become worse off than him: ridiculed, semi-intelligible, and full of shame. Except now we're old with a mouth full of brittle enamel, little sympathy, and no speech pathologist.

Floss doesn't put dentists' kids through college. A roll of floss could be free if we all started walking into our dentists, recycling the container, and asking for a new one. Find it in your budget and schedule to prevent a miserable toothless existence; it's hopefully no more than $10 per year.

Now, I understand that flossing after a decade of neglect might cause a bit of bleeding, discomfort, and the realization that we suck at taking care of ourselves. I understand that it might even add a whole two minutes onto our post-pornography bedtime routine. So yes, there are some barriers there. But compare having teeth to not having teeth for a second. Teeth maintenance is a short-term need with long-term implications.

I have prepared a step-by-step on how to master flossing.

Step 1: Purchasing floss. If we can't begin the recycling floss-containers movement then we'll have to beg a local dentist for floss or buy it at the store. Put it on the bathroom counter near the sink. Floss is not just a bathroom ornament to impress women who walk into your house accidently! If your current floss has accumulated bathroom grime (aka: shit dust), this is a sign that you are under-flossing.

Step 2: Using your floss. Remove the hygienic safety strip and carefully (it comes out fast and can't be put back in) remove enough floss to wrap around the preferred fingers three or four times. Pull the floss tight, but not too tight or it will snap, and run the length of the floss through the gaps of each tooth. Don't forget the back ones. Consider gravity with regards to long term build-up and make sure to do a good job on the backs of the bottom front teeth.

Step 3: Floss safety. After neglect, the initial thrust through the gaps can lead to lacerations. Your gums are that of a weakling, sir. With sustained effort, gums become resilient—gums are a metaphor for life. Now, like sexual intercourse, it isn't good enough just to go in and out with the floss and be done with it. Stroke the floss up and down along the inner wall of each tooth. This lets you clean the teeth individually and offers some degree of wrap around.

Step 4: Disposing of your floss. Your gums will probably bleed. It could be decades of neglect. In the unlikely event that you are having a sleep-over with a new girlfriend (though she will certainly be impressed that you flossed), you should probably try to hide the fact you are now bleeding from the mouth—this is especially unsexy. That piece of string is technically bio-hazardous. Placing it in the garbage is the commonly accepted practice.

I really don't want the young men of the world to lose their teeth. We risk becoming sexless rejects who people struggle to look at without recoiling in pity and disgust. To all those people living with tooth decay, sorry I didn't write this book earlier. Go talk to a dentist, no matter how bad it is; they might be able to help. Happy flossing!

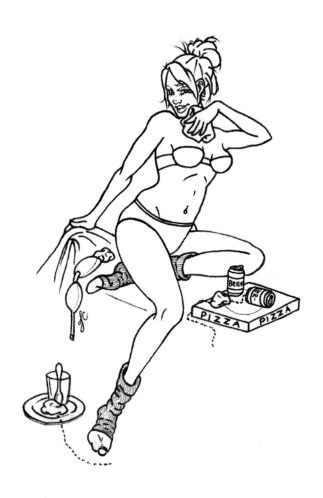

2.

Sex Before Supper Time:
Hygiene and Other Bad habits

Despite the short-term benefits of sloppiness, the purpose of hygiene is obvious to most. The un-fuckable male neglects hygiene in exchange for additional masturbation time. He also enjoys financial savings on cleaning supplies and personal products. Bathing, grooming, and cleaning may seem like chores, but that is only because they are. Home maintenance is a major part of manliness. Keeping your shit tidy is critical to getting fucked and loved.

Now, our mothers will never pick up our pizza boxes, soda bottles, and underpants ever again. She never should have in the first place! But she loved us just enough to stop a masturbation den from becoming a disease-infested cave full of ants and crusty tissues. Bless her for trying. Be sure to tidy up, unless your destiny truly is shlubby.

Despite some men's isolated, masturbatory, and repugnant methods, one-in-ten-million nerds invent a successful widget. In turn, that nerd king saves the rest of the nerds from persecution through tech-employment. Unfortunately, that single nerd's success is what justifies the other nerds' delusional lifestyles—lacking in basic hygiene, fitness, and social skills. The average dude requires a diabetes diagnoses, heart failure, divorce, or breakdown before he realizes his needs to change shitty habits. Isolation makes preventing health crises infinitely more difficult—no one is around to help. When men start suffering skeletal, muscular, heart, or rage problems, they are past the point of health prevention. Intervention is required. Isolated men risk fucking their lives up before thirty and that's mostly just a frame of mind. Gluttony is a hollow victory over giving up at life. Sadly, many of these self-aggrandizing, horrifically entitled, vampire-wannabes will become engineers, surgeons, or respected StarCraft professionals while remaining physically/emotionally inept for the rest of their stunted and lethargic lives. The only upside to staying this way is that death by elemental exposure is improbable, and they will never become important enough to murder.

The opposite of nerd-filth is trades-guy-filth, which can be equally (if not more) disgusting. These are industrious and hard-working men. These guys aren't slouches or necessarily stupid. If shlubby dudes hate on the trade's lifestyle, they're jealous, physically weak, *and* practically useless. For a cola-crushing gamer-type, this is a lose-lose attitude of other (very helpful) men in society. Jealousy doesn't make anyone look like a shining beacon of sexuality or confidence. It makes us look like insecure intelligencia and puts us in a shitty hypocritical ivory tower full of sperm-filled tissues and take-out containers.

Never the less, the men who get dirty in their daily work can still demonstrate poor hygiene despite their awesome productivity.

Working men can have great back strength, which is a major plus in the sack (Pro tip: work the hip-flexors), but lack social finesse. This lack of social finesse (in both male subtypes) limits a man's ability to have frequent, consensual, not-paid-for sexual interactions. Women are unlikely to strip a man out of concrete-matted Carhartts, sweaty underpants, and steel toed boots while he reeks of cigarettes and has dirt under his fingernails. Heavy industry is full of masculine overcompensation and lacking hygiene. Regardless of their rough social skills, the men of heavy industry still have a need for relationships and tenderness—or getting pussy, as they'd prefer to call it. That tiny spark of repressed romantic sentiment is his key to success. If these men couple strength with emotional vulnerability, they're on their way to being extremely attractive.

Shlubby men in isolation have significantly worse odds than active working men in achieving a sexual partner. It is the virtue of his practical skillset, the maintenance of his body, and his mindfulness of emotions which will help him stand out. Therefore, the advice below caters to men who are closer to sexual success—shlubs have a long way to go. I advocate for sex before supper during the week. This is how to go about negotiating sex Monday-Thursday within a pre-existing relationship.

Step 1: Pause before homecoming. Before you walk in the door, think about how your day went. How would you like to spend your evening? The likelihood of having sex is based on homecoming behaviour. Sports shows and a six-pack of beer, or a reasonable diet, a tidy environment, and a mutually relaxing night? A small pause before homecoming gives you time to reflect on how you are feeling and how your spouse might be feeling. This way, you will come home more mentally collected, which is essential to sex before supper. Also note that you can have sex before supper *or* beer with the buddies after work. You can't have both.

Step 2: Avoid that "how was your day" shit. You will find yourself listening to or giving unsexy complaints if you jump right into that. Instead say, "I love you; it's nice to see you," and then go straight to the bathroom for your post-work hygiene routine.

Step 3: Get a bathroom music device. Put on your favorite music, and make your post-work bathroom routine a special part of your day. Try a very hot shower to stimulate the skin followed by a quick blast of cold water to get the blood moving. Brush your teeth, floss, and apply deodorant.

Step 4: Put your dirty clothes away. Tidy up the room and make the bed. This is setting the stage: a candle, a flower, a chocolate, or any simple surprise will dramatically increase the odds of sex-before-supper. The point is that you are clean and your environment is tidy.

Step 5: Return to the kitchen. Go to your sweetheart and help her set the stage for dinner, like you've set the stage for bed (this might include any number of domestic chores). After you've prepped dinner and cleaned up a bit, whisper, "I'm going to have a quick nap before dinner. Would you like to join me?" This is a win-win. You either get a nap and wank, or in a best-case scenario you get a fuck and a blowjob. At this point, it is very important that any cooking elements are turned off and that the children are fully distracted.

She might not always join you, but don't stop flirting with your spouse. Keep trying. When your darling *does* join you, anything is better than nothing. A quickie, a minute of kisses, or an enjoyable cuddle is all worthwhile sexy progress. Who knows, a brief moment of endearing tenderness might lead to the magical morning blowjob. If she does not join you, a twenty-minute post-work nap will improve the likelihood of being more alert during the more traditional hours of fucking.

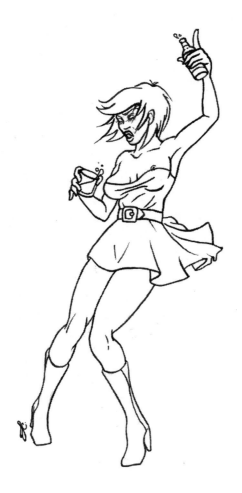

3.

The Dance Floor Man-Post

It is likely that you are (or have been) a dance-floor man-post. These are the guys who root themselves to the middle of the dance floor and bob their heads all night, just hoping they get noticed. Frankly, nothing is less noticeable. They are virtually invisible to women and become volatile because of it. Getting by on handsomeness, nice jeans, and bulky biceps is underselling man's all-around awesomeness. Maybe there is another dance floor man-post standing next to him bobbing *his* head offbeat. These dance floor man-posts are everywhere, packing the peripheries of clubs across the world with pervy moves and creepy stares. Don't let these guys validate you into not dancing. The dance-floor man-post can also be identified by double fisting domestic lager. His distinctive beer curls accentuate his arms, which distracts the on-looker from his thrusting pelvis. Looking around, you can easily notice a third dance floor man-post behind you, and a fourth attempting to bump-and-grind some woman half his size. These men will be wondering simultaneously who is going to be the first talk to that girl. Any girl, really.

Three drinks in, his hips begin to swing and false confidence creeps in. At five drinks, he starts a fist pump routine during the chorus. At six drinks, he's become convinced that he's the best goddamn dancer in this joint—and all the mother fuckers better watch out! At seven drinks, he'll become super possessive of a woman he's never met before. Finally, at 10 drinks, he's prepared to defend that woman from all the other dance floor molesters just like him. These nightclub superheroes (aka: douche bags) start fights over bullshit, and conveniently opt not to remember it. Thus he avoids consequences, lacks integrity, and is more likely die lonely. Note that this problem can be prevented if all men displayed mediocre dance moves. Fact.

Granted, there is no cure for terrible dance moves, but have you forgotten that you are a man? You do as you please and that includes dancing poorly! Bad dancing shows everyone how fun you are, and that you possess at least some sliver of genuine self-confidence and humor. Lousy dance moves help avoid cocky mistakes because you are already kinda silly. Dancing and sexy fun times are related but not guaranteed. Dance increases social magnetism and interaction. Admittedly, the drunken dance floor man-post is more likely to get fucked than, say, a wimpy wallflower (both non-dancers). However, wallflowers have some advantages in that they can avoid conflict at the expense of not meeting new people. Too many dance floor man-posts think nightclub molestation is the purpose of dancing. No. Wrong. Women everywhere agree that dancefloor molestation is gross and downright rapey. Confidence and dance skills are earned over time. Note that man-post and wall-flower will be out-performed every time by the happy guy dancing.

Dance floor man-post syndrome has a simple remedy:

Step 1: Smile. It's dark and dizzying on dance floors. Happy teeth stand out. This encourages the whole room to have fun. Talk with other dudes and establish a sense of safety for yourself. Other dudes might be haters, especially when your dance moves impress ladies. Note that and move on. Men will hit on the woman you've been dancing with. Fuck it—whatever, keep dancing! Be alert for when hostility and jealousy culminates in a need to duck. Douche bags can manifest violence and medical emergencies; use your man-senses to dodge aggression early. In a pinch, anticipate a shove and a sloppy right hook. Avoid participating in nightclub violence by using distance and appreciate metal detectors. Out-perform the competition by using caution, composure, and by making it known how you boogie. Contrast yourself, in the positive, with douche bags without condemning or antagonizing them. If a woman is into you, she will smile back at you and sustain eye contact. Though this is not a guarantee of anything sexual, it can be taken as a cue to say hello.

Step 2: Don't dance with backs. If you find yourself dancing with a woman's back, you are probably being intentionally ignored. Advance to the penis-to-ass dance routine (or bump-and-grind) at your own peril and potential criminal indictment. Should she promptly wheel around and smack you in the mouth upon you touching her ass, she would be within her rights. A smack indicates 'fuck off' permanently. Any groping whatsoever is a sexual assault, so move on. She is not a bitch for rejecting your sloppy ass. Rejection can escalate into disgust, she will hate you for being molested and disrespected. The dance floor molestation approach is for fuckos and perverts who lack basic communication skills and social finesse.

Step 3: Face time. Squaring off is the proper non-verbal method of approaching women on dance floors. When face-to-face, you'll be able to gauge her response to your sexy dance moves. As the sweat rolls down your back, the two of you might sync up. Her expressions will cue you to whether you'll be dancing all night or just for a few minutes. These expressions might include sustained eye contact, laughing, proximal advancement (touching), or flat out rejection. If you wind up dancing together for the bulk of the evening, enter phrases like, "My name is, X" "I'm-a get some water, do you want some?" "Can I meet your friends?" "I like your smile." Avoid comments about employment, living arrangements, or your salary.

Step 4: Up close. The most important connection is made through the frontal embrace. Wait until she reaches for you then move in close—mind your toes and her shoes. You are now cheek-to-cheek. Just sway to the music. In North American bars, it is likely she's going to lead the dance by essentially humping your leg. Don't get too fancy with the footwork at this point, just let her hump your leg while you lean back and try to keep rhythm. Due to the amount of sweat generated from the physical closeness and your rising erection, this state cannot last long much longer than an hour. If you are kissing like a pair of sloppy Rottweilers, or have a mutual urge to do so in private, start with phrases like, "you are really turning me on right now," "I live close by, if you'd like to uhh, have sex?" "Wanna check in with your friends and then maybe head back to your place?" "Can I get your number, I'm…we're… you're kinda drunk and I'm thinking we could put this off, till my dick actually functions properly…I really don't want to suck at sex any more than I already do." Rejection is guaranteed and perfectly normal, that would be a population catastrophe.

In the clubs, if the situation is flipped and you find a woman seeking you out for sex, you have an amber light for some sex tonight. This ass-to-penis (rather than penis-to-ass) dance routine is a whole 'nother level. This woman is temporarily aroused by alcohol, possibly attached, and probably capable of more sex acts than you can imagine—or just harmless a flirt. Basically, she is awesome.

But take note of how irrelevant you are to her equation—rejection is pre-determined. You could be anyone, barring only our hygiene and her prejudices. Have a condom prepared for these moments. Don't expect anything fancy and beware of dramas; just be safe and be happy about it as a form of delightful romance. Her possessive boyfriend (who her girlfriends hate) is out of town tonight, so don't leave any evidence that you have been inside of her. Also, be prepared for an emotional post-coitus, an immediate departure, and certainly no breakfast.

Now, for those wimps too terrified to step onto the dance floor: not dancing equates to being boring sexually and a cowardly man. You danced and skipped as a child. Now do it again, you rigid fuckhead. I swear, one day you will find yourself alone at a wedding or festival and that dance floor (which offers a wealth of togetherness) will haunt you. Your only refuge from this emotional isolation will be to surround yourself with other lame wallflowers too stupid to recognize that dancing is fun. As you and the other ugly bachelors sit (stupidly gaping at all the happy people dancing) enjoying that shared feeling of resentment, bitterness, and wishing you were someone else, realizes that you've done this to yourself, fucko. While the ugly bachelors validate each other's insecurity with alcohol and grunting, nothing can hide their ineptitude and need for change from the bridesmaids. Take the first step, put some fun into it.

Happy dancing.

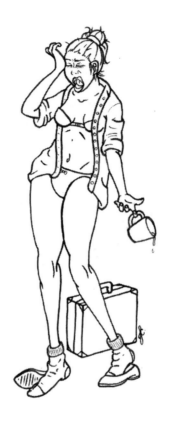

4.

Get Some Sleep, You Ugly Troll

Nothing says manliness better than vigor and alertness. Too many dudes spend hours on the internet or television watching bullshit late into the evening. Some men level up in online video games, while others obsessively scan the newsfeeds. Some gamble and masturbate like their cocks will fall off tomorrow. Sports and fantasy league football teams are a good social outlet, so long as it doesn't impact sleep. Some guys toil in the garage until after midnight, and a rising population desires endless late night entertainment from YouTube and Facebook until sleep becomes physically compulsory. This late-night monotony and boredom will impact our sex life—in the unlikely event that a sex life exists. It also affects our ability to accomplish stuff.

One thing men are famous for is doing stuff. When we find that in the morning we must begrudgingly drag ourselves from bed and desperately assess the coffee situation before anything else, we have a sleep problem. When our alarm is set to allow maximum sleep and minimum preparation time, we have a sleep problem. If we consume cold, unsatisfying breakfasts in less than three minutes (or skipped entirely), we have a sleep problem. This problem will result in crappy lunches in microwavable packages and evening binge eating. Worst of all, if we rush the morning, we miss the best time to have sex. If we don't sleep, we haven't got any time to whack off in the morning, and that is probably the largest part of our sex life.

Without enough sleep, we neglect essential morning activities (like sex and flossing). We'll be out the door in such a rush that the long-term impact of a shitty sleep schedule seems more manageable than the traffic jams. Our morning rush results in countless stained shirts, numerous morning blood-pressure spikes, and being an insufferable asshole. Upon arrival at work—assuming we are employed and have a safe place to sleep—it is virtually impossible to be genuinely pleasant. Meanwhile the peppy, sexually successful people are annoying as hell, all because you believe five to six hours of sleep is good enough.

We know we need more sleep, but the loving glow of computer screens feels like daylight. The extremely manly ones who have said "I'll sleep when I'm dead" are idiots. A dude can die from fatigue. Fatigue is a great way to drive your car into on-coming traffic or fuck up a machine-related operation. Tragedies such as these will, can, and do happen. Too often a young man's obituary reads, "He was just starting to turn his life around when suddenly..." Accidental change happens. Injuries can be prevented by foresight and education, but also good sleep. Life is an ongoing, day-to-day, work-in-progress that is always rebuilding. Life happens daily with every sleep.

Without sleep, we don't think as well. We risk severely compounding that thought-distortion with drugs and alcohol. Our mental health breakdown cannot be qualified until we have one. However, three days of late night boozing, a couple conflicts with friends, and an accidental injury will make happiness really difficult. Commit to sleeping; it's like a relationship with our future selves.

Men are creatures of action. Though procrastination can lead to making more thoughtful decisions, we cannot turn back the clock on our daily sleeping needs. Nine relaxing hours in a comfortable and safe bedroom is a blessing. Bedroom time is a damn good way to unwind, have sex, pray, write, chat with someone, make models, design cabinetry, tinker, trim toenails, water plants, clean the windows, or play with Lego—whatever. If you have a bedroom, use it for fun as well as sleep.

The electronic alarm helps us gain daylight productivity in exchange for nighttime hours (aka: lonely masturbation time). We fuck best when we are well rested and sober. Odds are that we are more sober during the daylight; therefore sex is an ideal daytime activity and does not necessitate sleep loss. Think of alarm clocks as accommodating a morning sex life (with yourself). Sleep deprivation inhibits overall success; it shows in our face and impacts our aesthetic vitality (you are uglier). When we don't sleep, we become lethargic and less responsive. Inside of relationships, to sustain a sex life, our sleep cycles need to align with our partners in order to consolidate mutual energy reserves. Less sleep means less energy to fuck later, it's like cause and effect.

Without lots of sleep, regular emotions become more difficult to manage. When stress creeps up on us, we unconsciously begin using (potentially) shitty methods of coping with it, including staying up late in restless contemplation or internet numbness. Of course we feel lonely at three in the morning! Participating in late-night internet consumption just reinforces the isolation, especially when we wake up at eleven a.m. every day.

So, how do we fix this? Meh,

Step 1: Identify what is keeping you up. Smoking weed and playing video games? Got stress on your mind or anxiety late at night? Does your partner like to cuddle too much and are you irritated all the time? Are you whacking off six times between 11pm-2am?

Are you worrying about your future? Have you been doing lines of cocaine all weekend? Maybe you're just like everyone in North America and just completely over-fucking-stimulated, dreadfully under-employed, and mysteriously addicted to sugar and salt?

Step 2: Acknowledge it as kinda a thing. Life is not ideal (it's a fucker) and your body suffers because you suck at being kind to it. How long do you expect your body to out run your mind? Not that fucking long! You could ignore your body forever and then just die. Having a very active brain and a miserable physical body is a depressing way to live. On the other hand, men who appear physically fit can be notorious for ignoring mental health problems— until they explode in abusive chaos. Fact: we are always emotional but we don't have to become volatile. Sleep helps us manage our daily emotional upsets. Being angry is easy when we are exhausted. Anger is the best way to compound our problems. A good night's sleep can bring down a temper and spare everyone our volatility. This does not mean we must invalidate our frustrations. If we feel shitty often, that is a very important thing to address. Applying some discipline, with regards to sleep, can be a first step in the process of making an ally of our minds. Our parents, coworkers, pets, children, and spouse will distance themselves from us if we become volatile too often. Sleep helps us to maintain balance by giving us the energy to handle life's stronger emotions.

Step 3: Make a sleep plan. A plan becomes a schedule. A schedule becomes a pattern. Imagine taking an hour to get ready for bed and an hour to leave in the morning. Something as simple as that will outline our sleep needs. Sleep should not have to be a luxury we trade for technology. Nobody is special or exempt from the biological demand of sleep. Use that man-brain, do a little math, and figure out when to get ready for bed. Train that inner child and send him to bed on time. Staying up late transforms us into awkward, apathetic grouches. We're liable to watch far too much porn, become filthy, and remain isolated. If we sleep more, we'll instantly become less of a target for social mockery.

Step 4: Enjoy your extra time. Oh my goodness, can you imagine having a full hour to do as you please before bed and in the morning? Gee whizz, you might be able to have a sex life again, or do a bit of exercise, or learn to read good. The internet, the television, your level 90 wizard, and your hot rod are nowhere near as important as your total personal health. Get out of bed each day and eat your breakfast calmly. Sip your beverage of choice in your kitchen chair. Sit and think and breathe. Perhaps have a light and thoughtful conversation with someone that you live with. Now that you have a sleep schedule, you might manage morning pleasantries better and possibly tolerate traffic.

Get to bed.

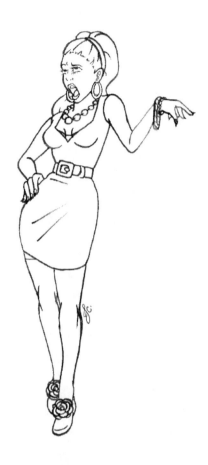

5.
Smarten Up by Shutting Up

Ever been in an argument that was pointless and irritating? Maybe it's a recurrent argument, or one we've had with ourselves every fucking day since puberty. This seemingly endless conflict could last for hours, days, months, or maybe until the day we fucking die. Even my dear grandfather harboured some conflict with his wife right up to the moment he died. As grandma held his hand in the last moment of his life, she asked him to wait for her in heaven. My grandfather's reply was simply, "I won't be there." "I won't be there" were his last words to comfort Granny while he died. Not "I love you." Not, "Thanks for all the support." Not, "What a beautiful life we've had together." Just, "I won't be there." Sure, it's the abandonment of their life-long religious agreement and the flat rejection of Granny in their life hereafter, but it's also hilarious.
She was dating within a year. Isn't that great?

Granny was (and arguably still is) a nag, I'm told—she's downright delightful with her grandsons. Have you ever wanted to end a relationship because of too much nagging? Or through force-of-nagging behaved responsibly because it was clearly for your own good? Or found yourself yelling profanities to drown out your spouse while simultaneously being very confused? Answering yes to any of these questions suggests a lack of perspective. This is the gravitational orbit for being a self-centred and emotionally numb douche bag.

It may sound ridiculous but our behaviours have a direct effect on other people. Understanding this principal makes having supportive relationships possible. There is no short-cut to over-coming vulnerability. In relationship development sex is an after-thought. Sex improves only with time and experience; begin by recognizing the importance of validating non-verbal and verbal communication. Close friends will be impacted by our shitty behaviours. For example, we might think that eating burgers, binge drinking, and barfing doesn't impact our relationships, but it does. This communicates to the outside world (including yo' mama) that we have a significant character flaws. Observers will inevitably interpret our behaviours wildly differently than we'd prefer. Masculine overcompensation (such as stupid risks and bravado) is hilarious in fail videos but absolutely fucking insane. Driven by aggression, overcompensation makes otherwise very boring men temporarily the king of idiots. I'm surprised there isn't a diagnosis for self-destructive man antics.

Men's words can be easily misinterpreted even when they aren't being loud-mouthed ignorant pricks. Use words carefully. Speak less. Accepting some flaw is a lot less stressful than hiding it with pride. But because of man's extra special emotional stupidity and lack of creativity, misunderstandings happen often. Communication becomes even worse when we get agitated, defensive, and chirpy. Detecting distress is easy for people who are close to us, so it's never necessary to yell at a friend, they can help us in a crisis if we ask. Outside of our social circle, however, our body language is what communicates our aggression levels. When triggered in public, just breathe, listen, and respond—try not to react. Everyone knows what it's like to be around an upset and hostile male. Men can become mean, scary, and threatening. Good luck getting healthy happy relationships with that much pride to protect. What we need today are men who are able to listen to what the community needs from them. Anger can be channeled positively, but it takes effort, which begins internally by becoming aware of our impact on the world around us—listening.

Young men are commonly found out at night binge drinking. Merry times were had at a rate hopefully higher than 90% fun. That 10% of not-fun needs proper calculation, however. Men need to learn the lessons of reckless men in order to prevent fucking up themselves—you're welcome. Otherwise, to keep our mediocre relationships alive, we'll be forced into conversations about reconciliation. These conversations will be highly emotional. If we improve our listening skills, conflict resolution will be far less tedious and angry. Nagging saves lives but frankly our listening skills make us very divorceable. When nagging (which we'd hoped would work) fails to change us, we've failed at an isolated strategy. Failure is upsetting but there are many routes to success. Failure only feels bad in the short term; setbacks in recovery/success are expected—don't get additionally hurt in the process. No man wins right out the gate and some men's setbacks really fucking suck. But life becomes longer when we set emotional milestones of success and failure, because those moments change us. If we can honour change, we may find more happiness and avoid future injury.

Anyways, failing is bad, right? Maybe not. Failure indicates trying. It is our negativity bias that is triggered to grasp tightly onto mistakes and never let them go. Negativity bias is useful in boxing, it teaches us how not to get punched in the head. But in our ambitions, navigating our flaws and overcoming our mistakes is part of our grand lesson and our core strategy. Trying and failing can reinforce doubt if we let it. Thus men become emotionally resilient by learning to rebuild their psyches and confidence, or they continue to hide. If we can't listen to the truth about our stupid behaviour (and respond accordingly), we become jerks at the expense of others. This is not a winning quality for togetherness.

The underdeveloped man-brain seeks to preserve its short-term self-image at the expense of long-term happiness. That is called insufferable pride. It invalidates other people's right to live and speak. By not listening, or by trampling a conversation with defensive crap, men ignore (obvious) personal problems, and the unhealthy long-term implications of rejecting others.

Unfortunately, one quality of togetherness is that if one person selectively forgets his lapse in sanity, the other person remembers. Any stupid pattern that friends know but we ignore is a shitty pattern. Friends informing friends about their boundaries and concerns is totally legit healthcare intervention. Hopefully, our friends can help us and forgive us, before we really fuck something up. We don't always get an opportunity to sort it out after we've fucked it up. Sometimes we don't get another chance to talk. We miss chances when we don't listen. A pattern-jackass knows what it feels like to be stonewalled by an old friend.

Trying to banish life's catastrophes into the darkest caves of our mind won't work forever. If we try to push out what we naturally feel then we will numb ourselves to other emotional options. Wishing away pain is a terrific strategy in mass prayer but on the individual level, it requires discipline, direction, and the ability to listen to criticism. Happiness can be measured in increments of change. Life's bumps are moments of change. Honour that shit. (Pro tip: seek good council).

Avoiding the consequences will lead to stupefaction and isolation. We learn nothing by ignoring others. We also lose the compliments that come with improvement. Everyone is worthy of supportive and healthy relationships—even ourselves. To get there, however, we've got to get co-operative feedback regularly. So shut the fuck up and listen to the critics, and that nagging inner voice. Having health positive relationships with friends is a great place to start.

Severely flawed men are completely emotionally dependent on women. They use women to pick up their ego from the dirt. She didn't fuck up his shit, it was his immature friends. If it wasn't his friends, then he did it to impress them. But since his man-friends are not of the supportive variety, he is banking on some future woman to magically appear and help his wounded ass. She might become his only friend who will tolerate him in the morning when he's gotten a cold. That mono-dependence bullshit will strain any friend's ability to keep helping us get it back together.

Be uncomfortable around modern women—she pulls her shit together every day. We were trained by fathers (or not) who were trained by fathers (or not) in a philosophy of life and how to value women. But post-WWII (and father-less) romantic sentiments are not needed today. This is like saying a computer science degree from the seventies is a critical requirement for employment at Google. When the shock wears off and we've accidentally become middle aged, we'll realize that we can't just go back. Dwelling on trauma and the resulting bitterness won't help us get well and active.

Some simplistic advice might sound like "you need to make some changes in your life," or "smarten the fuck up, jackass." Guys, we need to tell our man-friends when we see them fucking up their lives. If everyone you know is dumber than you, then you may have to lead the non-stupidity movement in your neighborhood.

Supportive man-friends are invaluable in a crisis (or pregnancy), but it may temporarily exhaust relationships. Relying on friends in a time of need might require an apology or a thank you later. Never be too proud to apologize or ask for help. This will subsequently require listening to advice. We value our man-friends (or "homo-social lifetime partners of indeterminate sexual contact") for their loyalty and understanding. When we risk that relationship with a crisis, we should be thankful for the help and apologize quickly. Be prepared for an earful of man-advise or some smack talk—same thing.

It is a big mystery why spouses take so much shit from men. Even she, the elusive female, has her limits and non-negotiable executive orders. Her limits are unique to every relationship. Actively discover those limits by listening. Don't test them, they come quickly. Defensiveness and rationalizing of our stupid behaviour is a sure sign of divorce territory. At some point, important phrases like, "I'm sorry" and "It won't happen again" may fail to satisfy the rage or embarrassment our partners feel.

If (by some miracle) she stays, during post-apology time, expect hours of critique. Listen to it carefully! This is better than a cold shoulder. Depending on the severity and frequency of the fuck ups, intensive emotional processing will be required to salvage this dream of lasting togetherness. We become better lovers and stronger men by realizing the effect we have on others. In theory, we *are* able to learn from our mistakes before we fuck it up again, but this is not always the case. This is called learning from past mistakes.

Infidelity does not necessitate violence. She can leave any time she wants. Don't panic. The divorce and restraining order are permanent, but the feelings of misery, rejection, and regret are only temporary (theoretically). When we get angry during the process of dumping, we are blaming a person we cannot change and cannot control. The only person we can change and control is ourselves. Attempting to control a woman with words or actions makes a man a fucking loser who is especially afraid of being lonely. The inherent powerlessness and helplessness of divorce can trigger a man's anger. Using aggression denies the feelings of whom we've hurt. It pushes people away from us and isolates us further. New insight and growth are impossible to find in a state of rage. Not listening reinforces our partner's belief that we won't change. This makes it more difficult for us to change because we've lost her positive (nagging) influence. It is a hard case to win when we don't shut up and listen.

Here are a few tips on listening.

Step 1: Temper your pride. Fucking up is accompanied with a feeling of horribleness, a sense of shame, incompetence, and dread. You might be considering running away or hiding. You might even try physically fighting your emotional problem by assaulting someone. Stop before you hurt yourself. Just surrender. Emotional distress is not a life and death situation until you escalate it. Let yourself be emotionally crushed. You fucked up badly, your masculinity is now in question, and you've shown how you handle adulthood (not well). Don't make it worse by acting more like a child about it.

Step 2: Unconditional apology. Your actions can create a flood of emotions in your support network. She may be acting hostile and mean, but I'd wager that your actions have contributed to the conflict. You only make matters worse by adding anger into the conflict. What you are about to learn are likely legitimate complaints about the quality of your character. When you begin to discuss the issues of your stagnation and incompetence, be prepared for additional evidence that highlights prolonged underlying problems. Phrases such as, "This is the same shit that happened last Christmas" illustrate what is called pattern-jackass behaviour.

You might find yourself defensively yelling, "Damnit! I've already apologized for that!" During an escalating argument, be aware of rage symptoms such as eye twitching, dangerous driving, resorting to alcohol, heart-rate acceleration, chest pain, or bleeding from striking inanimate objects. Before the point of escalation, you and your partner need to take an argument-recess immediately. Once you've safely, consensually, and completely exhausted this uncomfortable emotional reckoning with your spouse, it is time for your unconditional apology.

Step 3: Recap the feelings. If you are going to speak, stick to how you feel about what happened. What feelings drove you to behave in such a way in the first place? What might have triggered you? How do you feel now that the conflict is over? Do you understand how your actions made other people feel?

Step 4: Restitution and forgiveness. Forgiveness feels great, but being forsaken also happens. You must learn to recover from rejection peacefully—it's totally normal. Being forgiven should not feel like you've gotten away with a felony. Forgiveness should be a release from the emotional bullshit that you've been feeling. It will take a bit of time for your confidence to return. Be very kind to yourself for the next few days, then you can more-or-less return to your usual self, wiser and more mature than before.

I learned this strategy from screwing up a lot. By the time you are done with this book, you will be ready to bounce back from pretty much anything. The challenge is those pesky feelings and stupid behaviours that accompany our desire for generational continuity (or fucking).

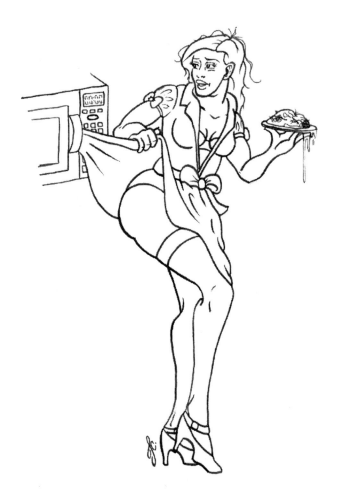

6.

Eat Shit and Die

This chapter is about death by dietary choices. It is time to get properly acquainted with food production. Meat was alive at one point. Vegetables and fruit grow out of the soil and require water. A single almond grown in California requires one litre of fresh water and there are ecological impacts to the over-fishing of tuna.

Fear not, for technology has made it possible to produce food in laboratories! Isn't that wonderful? Websites can inform us about agriculture, meat processing, and the magic of bio-engineering, but who wants free education when endless TV shows and processed meals are so cheap and easy to consume? Downloadable entertainment is far more fun than learning stuff—especially icky stuff like the slaughtering and raising of livestock.

Having a modern-day agricultural experience is unlikely. Today, the only livestock we encounter are cows at the side of a highway. Growing a tomato or any other vegetable is a quaint novelty reserved for hippy-farmers, new-aged mothers, the Amish, and environmental terrorists. Windowsills are allegedly capable of growing herbs and spices instead of just collecting plastic figurines, fast-food coupons, and stray recycling. Culinary television shows don't teach us about food production. They make us judge our own cooking as mediocre. Cooking shows have induced periodic fits of veganism and meal dissatisfaction in our population, but mostly they function as advertisements for the hosts. When we choose food documentaries instead of the latest sitcom, we will realize how food can fuck up our health. A shitty diet sets us up for medical problems that are largely self-inflicted and poverty related.

Instead of inspiring long-term dietary change, food documentaries are more likely to shame our microwave-dependency, which will inevitably lead us to culinary despair. How do men cope with feelings of culinary despair? That's right: emotional eating. Fuck it! Carry on eating whatever makes your mouth happy. We'll die before the world ends! All that really matters is that your food prep time doesn't take away from your sacred masturbation time. Don't think about what or why you eat, just eat whatever lets you return to the computer screen as quickly as possible. Bring a napkin for the crumbs and semen!

The Earth is finite, but are we helpless to stop its decline? Why bother—says the man with a limp dick. What? Give up trying? Get seduced by salty, meat-like by-products rather than a real life romance? Is consuming billions of chicken wings per year truly the natural course of life? Without culinary skills, men will be hopeless to sustain themselves healthily and therefore be less likely to sexually succeed.

Yup, I agree; things look bleak. If the planet is going to sustain this kind of population, food will either be factory and laboratory made, or we'll adopt hyper-localized growing. Instead of growing food, we are growing incompetent. We are helpless to feed ourselves a good diet and reluctant to change. Worst of all, we think it is someone else's responsibility to take care of us. Poisoning our bodies with five pounds of hot-wings and four lagers every Wednesday doesn't speak well for the long-term vision we have for ourselves. This is just a saucy, sloppy, sugar-coating of the feelings we have towards global helplessness— comfort food.

Men like solution-based problem solving, but why are we unable to solve our own lack of self-discipline with regards to diet? We can't even feed ourselves a reasonable and consistent diet! Seriously, how manly is that?

Go out and find a single edible plant. Community gardens don't count. I bet most men would poison themselves with what they find. Foraging is dangerous; don't do it without education. Preparing healthy meals, however, is sexy. Any woman will appreciate the use of good ingredients like avocados, walnuts, and spices. There is more to fruits and vegetables than just apples and carrots. Live a little, diversify the shopping list! For god's sake, try new things. One of the benefits of multiculturalism is that we import exotic foods; try some! We are so damn used to getting packaged, competitive, and machine-handled goods that we have forgotten how to cook.

The microwave was a terrible invention for obesity *and* for romance. Reliance on the microwave has contributed to an epidemic of television dinners and cholesterol. Nuked meals even come in their own trough. When we envision these kinds of presto-meals, we would like to imagine space-aged nutrition. More realistically, we think of overweight parents feeding their chubby children salt-rich slop because no one knows how to cook.

The downfall of the American empire won't be nuclear war. It will be disease, greed, gluttony, poverty, and heart failure. Obesity is a severe health problem with very harsh connotations. Cheap, low-quality food is passively sterilizing an entire evolutionary subset, and it will kill you too.

Here are a few simple steps to fix this conundrum:

Step 1: Identify emotional eating. Are you eating because you are angry or depressed? When you experience difficult emotions, are you prone to purchase sweets or salty snacks? Do you avoid going out of the house because you feel judged? All this stuff creates circular patterns of self-destruction through overconsumption. I'm only telling you this because I am genuinely concerned about your future-health, not because I hate you. Stigma can be the worst.

Step 2: Rate your cooking skills. On a scale of 1-10, how good a cook are you? If you are anywhere on the scale, that's a good start. A one means you have noodles and apples down pat. Excellent. You'll be ready for eggs and toast in no time. You are the only one who thinks you can't cook. You *can* learn. Why put yourself down when what you really need is to talk yourself up and learn some fucking kitchen skills? The fun thing about cooking is that there aren't many rules beyond "don't put metal in the microwave." Making meals is a creative task, and it might lead to sex. Like sex, with cooking you get to make it up each time. Trial and error is how babies learn, and babies are adorable when they are learning. Trying is endearing and women like that. Emulate children and keep learning. Release your inner mess!

Step 3: Buy healthy food. This one is painfully obvious, but you and your friends eat like idiots. You are addicted to sweet, fatty, and salty flavors. Who isn't? You have spent your life fluctuating between mild hypoglycemia and dehydration. Your shitty diet, which you designed upon leaving your mother's house, has set back your physical, mental, and sexual health. Every fucking day you are jonesing like an addict to match yesterday's sugar dose. Whatever you ate yesterday will drive your desires today. That is the definition of addiction. You are addicted to your diet. Substitute berries or raisins for sweets, and roasted nuts for the salty snacks. Do whatever works for you; get educated, but do it.

Step 4: Cook. What's the hang up? Shitty excuses abound for why not to cook. All of them are stupid and show a lack of sensible priorities. One excuse is that it takes too much time to cook. Well, keep eating shit and you will lose *years* of your life. How time efficient is that? If you avoid a healthy diet, you will risk that mid-life heart attack and that infamous limp-dick. Another excuse I have heard is that it is no fun eating alone. That is where you've got to start. Yes, eating alone never leads to sex, unless you count whacking off. Food is an amazing way to socialize, and once you have a few good recipes under your belt, hosting friends and lovers will actually become an option for you.

I'm not a nutritionist; I'm a jackass who cares about reducing the future costs of healthcare and having happier communities. Seek a dietician if you have symptoms of terrible digestion, but if you are like most guys, who never get help for anything until a crisis hits, the task falls strictly onto you. You can eat shit and die, or not.

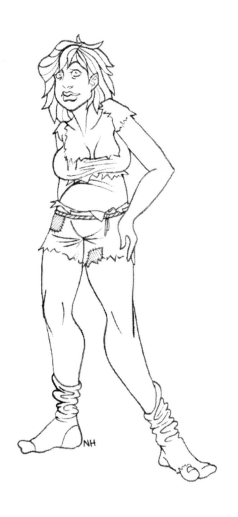

7.

Have You Ever Tried: Dressing Nicely?

Everyone dresses nicely from time to time: funerals, sentencing hearings, and first marriages. Try to have, at minimum, an annual function that warrants some fine attire. Maybe it's a comedy show, a fundraiser, or tapas and sangria at someplace fancy.

Guys can make dating more memorable by dressing up. Romance ain't a movie, and there's no script. It is spontaneous, safe, and sincere. Don't plan too much, and don't work off old expectations. On a date, be available by giving attention and listening—we simply add value when we dress nicely for the occasion. Act as if romantic moments are possible and they will be.

All dapper, like the embodiment of a personal sex god, he looks deep into her eyes and cues up for a kiss. Offering his hand, he gracefully rounds her mid-back and draws her close. Smiling and smelling her hair, he waits just enough to let the memory of this romantic moment solidify so that years later that same perfume summons up that moment all over again.

Holding lovers sweetly and tenderly is a wonderful lifetime accomplishment for masculinity. That loving acceptance within a relationship is a blessing. Exhilaration compounds with kisses, but does love require an orgasmic reflex? The emotional climax of our dick is an orgasm, which is followed by a physical feeling of peacefulness. It is sublime lying naked, post-fucking, and breathing in and out together. Aw, togetherness is important to us after all! Having sex tonight? Try beginning an even more intimate relationship by bringing explicit compliments into the bedroom. Compliments can start with clothing. Clothes say a lot about a man. With time, effort, and trust, we can get out of our clothes and into that sexy victorious lovers stuff. Confidence says we accept our flaws, but a sharp look says that we think highly of ourselves. In relationships, flaw development and change facilitation is key. Rather than use bravado, just dress nicely, because sex is a special occasion.

Sex is great but it is never a given. The best way to improve our sex potential is to care about ourselves. This can be interpreted by how we dress. When we encounter our ex-girlfriends, we hope to look semi-decent. These moments are impossible to prepare for, so it requires that we dress nicely often. When in doubt, be blunt and come as you are. It shows high self-regard and honesty. Good clothes are a good investment, even if they are from second-hand stores. Buy clothes of a reasonable quality and wear them for immediate improvement. Get in there! Thrift early, thrift often.

For dudes who aren't thrilled by second-hand stores, looking sharp is just more expensive, so get sale-savvy. There are lots of variations to men's fashion. Dust off that suit and plan to use it more than accidentally. Fashion purchases and a social life will impact positive social gravity. Don't underestimate that. Everyone passively judges what people wear—subconsciously—but this does not necessitate prejudice. Most of our lives are spent in denim to avoid confusion with sequins. Denim addiction not a big deal, but it benefits comfort and utility at the expense of zest.

We can't be on our A-game wearing denim. It is just too casual for our genius to be self-evident. Getting sized is a good first step. When opportunity comes a-knocking, there had better be an outfit to match our ambitions. Go discover cufflinks. Wear sexy cologne (but also just smell good naturally). Style your hair to the best of your abilities. Tattoos: show them, they're a big fashion investment. Bling out with rings. Get a gold and silver (coloured) watch. Pleats are for the super-hip but otherwise should be left in the prohibition era. If you do have pleats, wear matching socks. Shabby socks give away a sloppy suited male. Black work shoes don't count towards fancy attire. Get a splashy pair of dancing shoes for fancy parties. One pair of leather shoes of medium quality will suffice for most shindigs. Expensive shoes need Topy Soles—go see a local cobbler. Without them shoes wear out unnecessarily and let water in. 'I like your shoes' is a terrific compliment.

Handsomely dressed men get to talk to women in ball gowns and shlubby dudes don't—that's just fashion math. The thing about over-dressing is that no matter what the circumstances, we can always recover from looking too good. However, we cannot recover from looking underdressed, out of place, and like a slob. When we find ourselves wearing denim and plaid at the in-laws' New Year's Eve function the reason for our discomfort, is fashion.

So dress nicely. This is how to do it:

Step 1: Outfitting. Don't think you should be someone you aren't. The most important thing is that clothes fit. Frequently wearing our nice clothes will prevent the annual surprise of realizing we're getting fatter. There is nothing grosser than belly sticking out the bottom of a guy's T-shirt. Your pants must not be too small at the waist; it creates a muffin-top. Buy new pants. If all you have are black socks, black pants, a black pair of shoes, and a work shirt, buy a *black* belt, tuck your shirt in, and keep tidy in the face. A watch is a fine choice too; it's a symbol of diligence.

Step 2: Shopping. Women won't always dress us, but you don't need advice to look snappy. You're a man, do it yourself. If you are accustomed to a uniform and can't be bothered to make weekend fashion choices, that's shlubby. A cook's uniform, surgical scrubs, or coveralls for five days a week gives a man a lot of time to think about fashion. Chip in a little effort! Dull fashion highlights our mediocre creativity and externally brands us as average. Feel handsome by occasionally having something worthwhile to dress up for. This will require some shopping.

Step 3: Purchasing. Men in menswear departments are so funny to watch. Try not to be so awkward with the sales attendant—be enthusiastic. She is trained to sell clothes to women, and she doesn't care that you are lonely and single. Don't confuse flirting with upselling. Let them sell you stuff! Don't hold back! Try on everything! If the sales rep starts talking about matching colours, don't take offence— say yes! A sale at a retail store doesn't mean you get more for less, it means you spend more and get more. For the first few times, you will be annoyed with the expense, but the annoyance will fade as you get comfortable purchasing your own nice clothes.

Step 4: Partying. Have a social life. Look forward to something (like parties, ceremonies, or dates) so that you have a reason to get dressed up. Have, at least, an annual event on the horizon that requires that you dress up nicely. Fancy parties don't have to be amazing or expensive. Being well-dressed will make a date more memorable. Whatever events you're into, be it nightclubs or church sermons, our clothing reflects how we wish to be seen and our current outlook. Make a date to dress up for and follow through. Simple as that. Do stuff. Different types of outfits may be required.

When it comes to being nicely dressed, a lot comes from culture. There are no right answers to style. It is up to you to choose how you want the world to perceive you. This is called fashion. Fashion impacts your social gravity. Consider fashion conscientiously to understand how it influences your mood. Seek out a style that suits your happiest values and likeminded people will be drawn to you. This will help avoid death by denim addiction, mediocrity, and isolation.

By looking nice, life might feel more important. Eventually it might *be* more important.

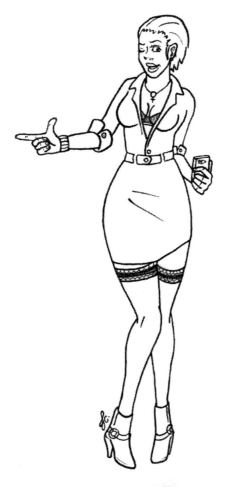

8.

Every Man Has an
A Game

At some point in life, we have displayed at least a minimal amount of potential. In that bygone moment, when we tried at life, was there an original moment of having our feelings hurt because of some kind of failure? Oh, those pesky memories. Flashback memories of our own failures indicate how we have learned to suck at life. Initially, we can attribute our shortcomings to trauma or abuse; unfortunately as an adult male, we are responsible for overcoming those issues, regardless of how much we blame external forces.

We all have those moments of wanting to give up and stop trying. Men are guaranteed to have moments of rejection, failure, and shame. Otherwise, it would mean we never tried anything. A man must calmly and knowingly fall into an emotional breakdown, not be ambushed by it. We don't solve problems by running away, curling up into the fetal position, or putting our hands through a wall. It's funny how drywall needs an unusual amount of fist-repair. Often we don't realize that our stupid behaviours create negative patterns that inhibit our A-game.

We don't just wake up one day with a dreadful sense of purposelessness. It builds up over a long time. That state of meaninglessness began when our failures drove us to stop trying. We unlearned fun or learned that the fear of failure was worse that the exhilaration of trying new things. It's a red flag when a man has tried less than two new things in any given year.

This doesn't mean you need to take a fucking pottery class or learn salsa (although those are valid choices). It just means that it is extremely good when men are curious about things beyond themselves. Having interests makes life interesting—and not just for Facebook. Having personal interests will make us less defensive when surrounded by cool people. Also, women might actually enjoy our company. By genuinely being interested in life, we stop sucking the life out of our friends and lovers. A man should be able to occupy himself with his own curiosity—more than just his dick. If spending an evening or weekend separated from our wives or girlfriends makes us uncomfortable, jealous, drunk, lonely, sleepless, or abandoned, then there's a problem. We don't embody a worthwhile person to come home to if we're that needy.

Put on the A-game. Try living again! There may be limitations, but work within them. Break old habits by trying, failing, and trying again. Try amateurism so that you will have stories to share with friends. This isn't a status update or joining hate groups. This is living with curiosity in the world. It shows that we are in pursuit of possibility and not stuck in a rut. Look back to childhood and recall the man you wanted to become. Go try! Don't lie or embellish accomplishments, just go out and do stuff. We screw up a lot more than we succeed—get used to it. Brag about resiliency and a commitment to life-long learning so that if we have sex eventually (which is doubtful), that person might really like us.

For those who are stale, here are some tips on becoming less divorceable:

Step 1: Have interests. If you don't have an interest that can be appreciated, people will fake their affection depending on their level of desperation. If you don't have interests beyond work, bromances, or entertainment, you are not interesting. Get curious about stuff.

Step 2: Articulate your interests. Should your interests be subjected to a severe amount of social stigma, be prepared to restrict your peer group or amount of disclosure. Examples of stigmatic hobbies include (but are not limited to) binge drinking, extremely nerdy stuff, gang activities, sexual objectification, religious zealotry, or politics. Barring that, you should feel able to discuss your activities with friends and lovers with some enthusiasm.

Step 3: Sustain your interests. A runner who exercises one week out of the year sets himself up for failure and injury. Dreaming of participating in an activity that you know will bring you joy is ill advised. Talking about doing a thing is not the same as actually doing it. Do it now and do it often. Nag yourself and make supportive relationship around your interests. Developing new patterns takes persistence. Change doesn't happen overnight but there is a big difference between a minor slip and a stagnation relapse.

Step 4: Do new activities. When you find that something isn't working anymore, find something new. Saying that you are interested in football when you haven't kicked a ball around for twenty years is foolish—go participate! When an activity repeatedly isolates you from human interactions (ie: video games), this hobby isn't transferable into social skills and needs re-working.

The point is to resist stagnation because it will permeate your relationships. Lacking passion transforms into monotony and crappy relationships.

At the point of divorce (or abandonment), you can become a rage-filled douche bag who blames his problems on someone else, or you can accept that you've been out of touch with your goals and become isolated.

I hope that you might reinvent yourself and bring that A-game back to life. Start with curiosity.

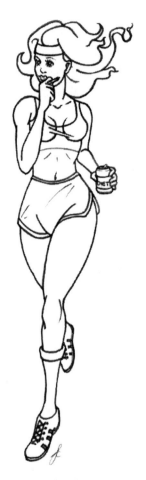

9.

Change is Unlikely, but You're Probably Half-Decent Anyway

Fact: nobody is coming to save us and make us happy. Despite being somewhat ugly, accident prone, and emotionally stupid, men are mostly good. We have sexual hang-ups, fear of rejection, supressed family issues, and we ignore old injuries. Nevertheless, we can frequently make ourselves smile and enjoy life's many pleasures. To get the most out of life (and prevent dying drunk and alone), a man must carefully weigh his stupidity against his kindness.

Let's assume clinical support services (like counselling and shit) is unaffordable or (stereotypically) that most men fucking hate the idea of seeking emotional help. Therefore, men are just blindly encountering thoughts of addiction, violence, suicide, numbness, and worthlessness without any guidance whatsoever. Therefore, men will struggle to identify their underlying problems: man's poor emotional vocabulary and stigma regarding weakness presents crippling psychological dilemmas. He can't articulate himself, so he doesn't know how to ask for help, and if he does, he will suffer emasculation from his male peer group. We have high tolerance for this kind emotional stupidity in men, so much so that men believe numbness, with intermittent explosions, is normal male behaviour.

It is a pity that stereotypical masculinity doesn't accommodate wholesale excellence for every man and his free expression. Telling our buddies about our life coach, spiritual healer, or guidance counsellor is unlikely because (despite it being healthy for the individual) it is in opposition to macho-masculine conformist stupidity. Unfortunately, because men have been trained to be emotionally inept, healthcare maintenance is somehow shameful among our peer group. Fuck'n hell, hey? You might be the only one who is actually trying.

We can't help being ourselves. Wigs, cosmetic surgery, and anti-aging products are not self-improvement. We get one face, one reputation, one life; don't fuck it up any worse. Shit, try making it better! Mistakes were made, but only fuck-ups quit. All the bridges are now officially burned. We forgive ourselves of our offenses, wrongs, and retaliations. Let go of that guilt. Hanging on to past mistakes will only make us feel ugly. We show our basic goodness by not giving up and evolving with the times. Part of that evolution is to recognize when to ask for help. Random binge drinking followed by deep and meaningful conversations with strangers is not counselling. It's just a minor emotional breakdown taking place in isolation from people who are able to help.

Contemplate how to live happily. Don't go too far into the future—we definitely aren't there yet. Matrimony isn't a green light to get lazy, not by a long shot. By pre-emptively embracing change, we begin relationships as (at least) a semi-decent guy. It is when a man becomes complacent that he needs an emotional shock to break his rut. Being dumped will suffice, but accidents happen. A divorce is a chance to improve just as much as it is an opportunity to crumple. It is an uphill battle to keep that penis functioning through alcohol, worthlessness, cardiovascular weakness, and old age. Staying active mentally and physically is what it takes to maintain our youthfulness. We all have strengths, but for the most part we don't use them enough.

Here are some steps to balance our strengths and weaknesses.

Step 1: Contemplate. Just think about it. At some time you have heard a nagging voice inside your head that said, "Damn you, you fucking loser. Get your shit together. Start doing something." That voice is your body and mind telling your consciousness that you are unhappy with your current state of existence—this can be very scary. Feel free to numb this negative, lifesaving voice with alcohol, mediocre sex, and illegal drugs. However, in those few sober moments, the urge to change will return accompanied by varying levels of rage and misery. You risk a repeating cycle: a strong desire to escape or change. Just think about what you want to change. No pressure, just think about it.

Step 2: Revert to old ways. Yup, you fucked it up. You tried to change and failed. So fuck everything! Never strive to change again. You failed, it sucked. All your friends know how badly you failed, and now you feel hurt and ashamed for being such a fucking failure. Stay inside for a few days. Curl up in a fetal ball and, when you are emotionally well again, revert back to your old stupid habits. Welcome to the realization of how important this change is to you. The anger and disappointment you are experiencing is a testament to how badly you wanted the change to stay. Your mother and your girlfriend are proud of you. But as a man, isn't it alarming how ineffective you are at controlling yourself? I hate to say it, but this is part of the journey.

Step 3: Try again. This time you should seriously plan for curveballs, stress, toxic situations, and major breakdowns. There are a lot of resources out there to explain change, but essentially, the manliest thing you can do is never give up (this is not the case in dating). Trial and error sucks. The more information you can get the better. Social support is critical. That is why isolated men like gamers, macho douche bags, and computer-programmers will die at forty-five from a lack of social skills *combined* with heart disease. If you operate in isolation, you are not going to change. With nothing to lose other than your own self-respect, you have nothing to gain. So put your pride into it and tell the world what you seek to become.

Step 4: Repeat. Change does not happen overnight. You are a half-decent guy already, so play life to your strengths. No one is going to do it for you. There might be a time when you reject everyone who you thought was a friend. There might be tears. At times, you will blame others and wish that all the bad feelings would go away. In time, dear friend, they will be resolved. You cannot fight against time (it's like gravity); you will lose. Regrets, setbacks, and disappointments are lessons learned, and only require temporary suffering. Change begins every morning and continues for the rest of your life.

You can, as many have before, live at 20% capacity. Your lovers and friends will advance beyond you. Only after a severe shock will you realize that men often live in denial and delusion. Self-improvement and openness is essential for long healthy relationships. Honesty is not a tool to enforce fidelity. It is how life can become more fun! Reduce the shame of being a fuck up by using blunt honesty.

Stay who you are and get even better. That is the goal.

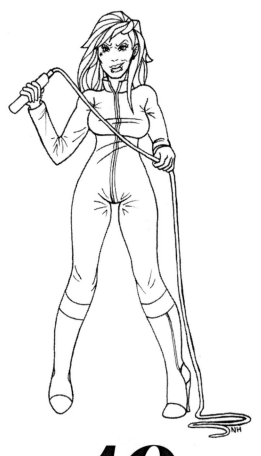

10.
Nagging Saves Lives

Men enjoy being nagged. It simplifies things because we don't have to think about where to improve. For centuries, men have used nagging as their primary preventative care strategy. In its extreme form, however, men can equate nagging with resentfulness. This is a tediously hypocritical reaction, gentlemen. It's like getting angry with a person who knows you really well when they give you good advice, like, "Take a deep breath and stay calm," or "Keep your eyes on the road, please." Naggers need not be hollered at or beaten off. Our tiny acts of misinformed rebellion against nagging can lead to insignificant victories at the risk of injury, illness, and rejection.

Many an' educator can go fuck themselves. Our spouse, family, and friends however should feel able to speak to us when our behaviours are reckless or dangerous. Becoming resentful when people try to help us just compounds our problems. We need to ask ourselves what we want, how we intend to get there, and if it is currently working. We can't expect to achieve a happy life without support, effort, and some change. Feeling nagged is a negative reaction to someone potentially offering help and encouragement. We need some nagging to help our masculinity take root and blossom—someone who cares and believe in us enough to give us some direction. We can't rely fully on ourselves; the hyper-masculine male is gunning for mediocrity, injuries, and isolation. He has strengths but his attitude about strength makes him a menace. When men are selfish, they isolate themselves. What we need from men is communication and co-operation.

Marriage, live-in relationships, and dating requires co-operation. Sexual relationships possess some degree of emotional and spiritual sexual intimacy—and a significant time investment. This is a rare type of relationships for a man. So when an important romance ends, is it that shocking that he might become suicidal after divorce? He may have expected the world from her. He was committed! He was doing it! Yes, all the way. Every day! Finally, one of the big guys. His sex life became the physical manifestation of everything he never thought he wanted: a baby boy! He fucked someone and she had his baby. And vice versa. You know it, I know it. It happened. In. A. Vagina.

But when he loses his relationship he goes back to having crappy support systems and an inept emotional culture with his buddies. She will probably recover from divorce more gracefully—but with added danger. When men get dumped they risk going into incredible anger—which is very bad for everyone. It takes a significant amount of time to recover from relationship loss, and enacting violence makes it much longer. As on-lookers, we have no fucking clue how to deal with men lashing out—there isn't a good way, just duck and run!

A relationship where we practice unquestioning emotional dependence will end with some kind of internal explosion. An unsatisfied spouse or a premature monogamy can end with feelings of failed expectations or that it was a regrettable waste of time. Resentment will pass. During relationship-loss recovery, direct the internal anger creatively, towards self-awareness. What are we seeking? What are we offering? How can we recover from this? When enraged, use distance, time, and oxygen.

In a divorce, we enjoy wealth dissection as well as misery. Becoming suddenly aware of long-standing warning signs also sucks. Don't blame the wrong person, try to take responsibility and stay calm. When she presses for divorce, her assessment won't be inaccurate. There are a lot of unaffectionate men who haven't bothered growing up yet. The tragedy here is that this is a common complaint. In divorce we risk losing half of everything and all of our sexual confidence (hopefully only temporarily). It can be avoided by validating her encouragement (aka: nagging) with active attempts at improvement. Thus, by pre-emptively trying self-improvement, we hedge our bets in future relationships. It would be a shame to get stuck with only our own nagging forever. Doubts and regrets; alone forever.

It's very easy to ignore problems when we are isolated. Lashing back is total shit-head behaviour when confronted with your short-comings. Giving abuse is worse than receiving. Abuse and violence comes through self-loathing and is the active devaluation of life. It is perpetuated by how we treat ourselves. Under no fucking circumstances does anyone deserve to be treated like how you treat yourself. No fucking thank you. Men can be volatile as fuck. Someone nagging is someone asking you to be kind to yourself. Your insistence on being an asshole to yourself is the problem.

Make good decisions for you, your friends, children, family, and neighbors. A long series of bad choices will leave you with no community, and that's a hard trend to reverse. Be seen striving for something, anything, so that the prayers of our friends, exes, and families can come true. This is the path to happiness and redemption. Too often by the time a man can fully realize himself, there isn't enough time to apologize.

Men fuck their lives up before thirty, and recovery is a bitch. For some reason many men feel obliged to follow a shit streak until an accident, injury, diagnosis, or divorce happens. For too many dudes, this is how they discover health maintenance. We shouldn't need to suffer a crisis to understand how to take care of ourselves. The key word here is prevention.

If we aren't getting nagged by our mother or wife, who is going to motivate us? Ourselves? How well has that been going? Every day gravity crushes our spine just a little bit more. Once we stop growing, we start shrinking and fattening up. Shabby habits will persist forever unless we actively try to change.

Be less divorceable:

Step 1: No one will save you. A woman is not the light of your life, your other half or the best thing that has ever happened to you. It is your job to save yourself from the long list of stupid shit. Your dangerously stupid, belligerent, defensive, and emotionally insecure bullshit is not a woman's responsibility. Accommodate gradual change. You can't afford a personal trainer or a home gym, so without a magical fucking personal journey (like this) you'll be stuck in fad-like happy-lifestyle efforts without a personal touch. Masturbation does not count as exercise or self-improvement. You're a sad and tragic joke if you don't realize that you are responsible for your response to life's adversity. This doesn't mean go it alone.

Step 2: Accept criticism. We're basically good but are often pricks. We're fat, ugly, under-achieving, over-stressed, under-educated, weak, rude, hostile, filthy, boring, stupid, and have lame interests (that nobody likes). We can also be a fucking embarrassment to our family. Those are insults. Criticism is different but still unpleasant. When we fuck up, we beat ourselves up even worse. People can't criticize us any worse than we insult ourselves. However, external nagging highlights stuff we hadn't considered fully. Over time, nagging will change us if we value companionship more than our rut. We can all see the benefits of being challenged by someone we respect. Acceptance will come; we are all kinda weird. Folks dislike the behaviours that negatively impact them, not us as a whole. Just breathe and listen to what people can tell you about yourself.

Step 3: Be stupid. It is less stressful. Being not-so-smart (even though we are) lets humility shine through. Everyone appreciates it when a man's pride barrier comes down and he listens to advice. He becomes a more interesting person when he is humbled by his character flaws before they bite him in the ass. Humility can lead to being comfortable within our own skin and maybe even facilitate a sex life.

Step 4: Be responsible. Nothing says, "Dump that man" better than him denying a problem and then repeating it. If you intend to continue as a fuckup, then you should end intimate relationships as soon as possible. Dump her fast, dramatically, and in public. Then, while getting exceedingly drunk, fuck a hooker, only to brag about it online later. This will terminate the relationship permanently through a negative learning environment. If that isn't sufficiently awful, after you sober up, call her immediately. Then, like a teary-eyed weasel, tell her you how sorry you are. Tell her that now, after that epic night of irresponsibility, you are ready to change. When she softens, manipulate her into coming over. Have a pretend-emotional quickie and make sure you get a BJ (as it might be your last). Get her to drop you off at the gym and don't phone her for at least a week. Then everything will be all better and she'll have forgotten everything about your fuckup. Right? As long as this woman puts up with your shit, repeat until you've both lost your self-esteem. In recovering from a relationship, the emotionally inept man might resort to abuse, fighting, stalking, suicide, murder, or harassment. Men must mitigate these emotions with support networks. Chill dude. Don't compound your problems. The more you resist nagging, the more you re-enforce your delusions of being awesome when really there is still a lot of work to do.

We can't hide an overwhelming sense of inadequacy forever. We need someone to help us be vulnerable, but no one will and we won't ask. O lonely, repressed, and helpless fucks. How did we get this way? Wouldn't it be nice to get some instructions? Reconsider nagging as a positive thing (Pro-tip: sustain a love life).

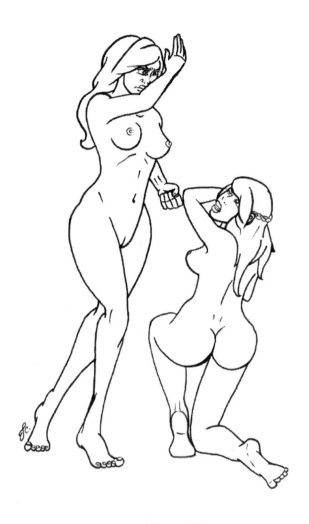

11.

Wimps and Jerks Don't Get Self Esteem

Wimps and jerks are the most devoid of self-esteem. Self-esteem is the placement of worthiness in one's self. It means respecting ourselves. Greater than respect, ideally we should also believe in ourselves. This, however, risks showing the world that we are actually trying which can be used against us by our stupid male peer groups. Men need to understand how they came to be who they are. There is no sense in over-compensating or being self-piteous. For better or worse, we are products of our environment and experiences. Accepting flaws is what puts us on track to finding self-esteem.

Being a weakling is unhealthy. For example, if a man's poor muscular development makes him unable to lift a bag of cement, gravity is going to hit him hard as he ages. Weaklings are welcome to validate themselves through having a great online personality (aka: working in technology) but at the end of the day if they are physically weak, that's bad. Sad muscular development can make a man a target for lethargy, fatness, and potentially staying at home a lot. A pathetic standard of fitness will drain our sense of self-esteem because masculinity requests some physical prowess. We might think that it is normal to be physically weak but that is only because it is so fucking common. This is one category (weaklings) which we want to resist. Without genius-level intellect, it is essential for men to participate in some medium-weight lifting. Without sustaining our musculature, we will get a noticeable stoop in our necks. Nothing says unsexy like failing to hold our heads up straight. Bellies will protrude and our faces will become pudgy and blotchy. This transformation has been forewarned by an inner nagging voice but wimps ignore it, and the physical effort life demands. Acknowledge big red flags, such as if your inner voice ever sounds like this:

"God, you're getting fat. Were you always that weak? I sure wish I could look like that guy in the store. Nope, that's never going to happen. Not for me. I can't change. I'm a worthless, aging, socially sidelined complainer that nobody wants to hang out with. Hell, I'll be lucky if I ever have sex again."

Get some help immediately if that's the case. In the unlikely event that we have a special woman in our lives, she will probably sugar coat our mediocrity and simultaneously reinforce it. This will make us feel temporarily relieved, but it won't solve shit. Make this a workable problem and just call it what it is: physical weakness.

As for the mean guys: you're jerks and I hate you. Everyone does. Bullies lack self-esteem just as much as weaklings. That is why bullies are so attracted to weaklings (they're both losers). Bullies tend to harbour some unresolved trauma (like abuse 'n shit) and have some legitimately sad excuses that explain their shit-head behaviour (often so do wimps). That is, if they've been court-ordered into therapy or fucked themselves up enough to realize a need for change. I'm guessing, however, that bullies don't tend to stay in therapy. The emotional rationale of men who inflict violence is baffling, but it is irrelevant to the victims and witnesses who now despise them. Bullies get isolated, impotent, and have massive waves of insecurity. They must keep life simple in order to maintain their emotional stability and zone of control—this includes bullying people into conformity. This common form of manliness is best dealt with by distancing ourselves from their bullshit. He believes that extensive isolation, hard labour, and grunting will stave off his daily addiction and anger. Rarely does he self-reflect outside of prison. These men are prime candidates for domestic violence because their emotional intelligence is below that of what is necessary to cohabitate with women. Verbal conflict is their preferred method of emotional defense and their desire to win can act as a bellwether for potential violence.

Bullies have extremely restricted comfort zones, and fear of emasculation worse than death. These men are conditioned to express only minimal amounts of feelings and tend to only emotionally bond with women. This dependency leads to a serious fear of sexual rejection. Since women are his only known emotional outlet, love-loss is scarier than a back injury. The restrictive masculinity of bullies accommodates mostly only polar emotions: anger and happiness. When he's sober, that is. Jerks feel powerless to improve their intelligence and they compensate by placing their self-confidence in their physical strength, status games, or risk taking. By using intimidation, bullies claim power, avoid feelings, and uphold their delusional male self-image. By being mean, they validate their only discernible positive quality: forcefulness. It is a scary task for a bully to get smart after years of angst and social marginalization. Mostly it's because everyone hates him and he has no support. Change can happen in two ways: consciously through self-reflection, or accidently through incarceration, injury, or death. Most bullies learn the hard way and don't recover quickly.

Everyone loves to see bullies fail—the harder the better. This is because we hope that he learns quickly from his irreparable injuries and becomes a better man. Nothing teaches a man a lesson like breaking bones or having an accident. If it takes a motor vehicle accident for a man to realize that life is precious, that's unfortunate. The problem is that he might hurt someone else in the process. Here's the mind-set of a douche bag contemplating change:

"You are such an idiot. I wish I could, but I can't. I can't change. God damnit! If I stayed in school I could have been a… I hated those teachers, I just don't understand math. If my dad hadn't been such an asshole, I wouldn't be in this mess. But I miss him. If my girlfriend hadn't acted that way, I wouldn't have had to… I'm sorry! I said I'm fucking sorry. Damnit woman! I'm so fucking angry with you right now. I could fucking kill that guy. I just want to get out. I'm leaving. I'm going for a drive. I don't know where. I'm just going. I don't know when I'll be back. Yes, I got drunk. Yes, I got stoned. No, I don't care. I hate this shit. Fuck this relationship. Fuck you and fuck your stupid friends. Fuck you. I love you. Don't go. I'm sorry. Fuck! You fucking bitch, don't you walk out on me!"

There is no limit to the intensity of this negative voice within the mind of a man in a rage. This state of madness is where thoughts of murder, suicide, and rape form. They are created by a lack of self-esteem. No matter where we are on this spectrum of wimps and jerks, we must know when to stop, admit that we've been fucked up for a long time, and be radically kind to ourselves.

Here are some tips on self-esteem. Start with self-worth:

Step 1: It changes. It's normal for day-to-day feelings of self-esteem to fluctuate. Sometimes things trigger us and we become less awesome in our mind's eye. We need to resist perpetual misery or recurring mediocrity. Self-esteem has peaks and valleys. This does not require going numb. Feelings of accomplishment compared to feelings of rejection have a direct correlation to your sense of self-worth. Misery and elation should both be temporary. Peppy be-happy propaganda is unrealistic, but so is lifelong numbness. The point is that feeling good about ourselves will improve the likelihoods of accomplishing our goals.

Step 2: Work on it. There are many ways to improve your self-esteem. Humans are never fully satisfied, so we are prone to this problem of wanting more. We are driven to continuously improve our environments and this makes self-esteem seem out of reach—overcoming this requires self-reflection. Everyone believes they can be better off, and therefore life is perpetually a work-in-progress. If we crumple and give up on self-improvement, we'll stagnate and increase the odds of dying alone. Small improvements are better than none.

Step 3: Brag. Don't make up lies, but consider getting some encouragement through bragging. This isn't a status update, this is telling friends about the cool stuff we do. Whatever your hobbies are, really get into them. Let yourself become fascinated with what you do, and share that enthusiasm with others. This has the benefit of helping you become smarter and being interesting in conversation.

Step 4: Positive self-speak. It's corny, but saying nice words to ourselves is a good thing. If you want, you can even try saying nice things to other people. Whenever possible, remember to be exceptionally kind to yourself. Our attitudes will change when we create positive environments for ourselves with encouraging friendships.

There is nothing sexier than a smart person with a workout routine. Wimps and bullies put too much stock in orbital facets of living. Strength and intelligence can exist simultaneously and are only two of the many virtues of masculinity. Temperance, kindness, and happiness are far superior to the malice and cowardice expressed by wimps and jerks.

You are more dynamic than you think you are.

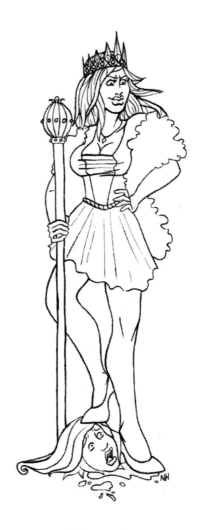

12.

Earning Things and Avoiding Hypocritical Entitlement

We are taught to think we're special, but really, are we? In a sense, no. An individual human life over a course of centuries isn't special. However, we are unique in some regards. Our experiential learning environment and excretions are one-of-a-kind. For example, right now unique bacteria are forming on the backs of our teeth and assholes. Each of us has a different smell in our toilet bowl. Our semen is a petri dish that scientists can't get enough of. The end result of our food process yields, on a micro level, a truly unique specimen. Men have a globally distinctive odour. The pattern of our body hair is unlike anyone else's. How we sneeze is also distinctive.

A man's experience is unique as well. Through life, we have made standards for ourselves and the world has taught us what to expect from it. This is a safe but ignorant frame of mind. Comfort is good until it changes or until our routines get burdensome. Change is good but slightly unpleasant. We can choose to remain unchanged but we can't rightfully impose our rigid standards on others. It compounds the stagnation. If composting and recycling is too much change to ask for, how can we be so condescending to anyone else who is just as equally unable to change?

In the workplace, in the streets, and in the bedroom, a sense of personal entitlement does not help build relationships. For example, just because we have an erection does not entitle us to its biological utility. A good life comes from the proficient use of the body and the mind. The dick is not the foundation of success and happiness. Sustainable sexual relationships, like a profession, are earned, trained for, and developed over time. Happiness and success come with many uncomfortable lessons, but we don't have to learn them all the hard way. Articulating lessons learned is a modern rite of passage. Short-term sex flings don't teach us anything about sex. Neither does getting fired before the end of the probation period.

Sex and work (both aid happiness) require effort. Apply some fucking initiative, jackass! Repeat sexual performances are like employment stability: they can benefit everyone. We learn a lot from a sex partner and we learn a lot from employment. When we lose our job, do we give up forever? No. The emotions of sexual rejection are just a temporary experience—accept rejection and move on. Get back on the horse and keep discovering life. It doesn't matter how many thrusts per minute, or how many hours we work. What counts is happiness and participation. This means enjoying the benefits of work, life, and our relationships. I hazard a guess that confidence in performing sex might seep into our leadership abilities. Being comfortable naked requires communication and vulnerability. So does leadership. To break out of hypocrisy, two virtues are essential: communication and vulnerability. Entitlement leads us to neither.

Once we establish a baseline sexual competency (which many of us haven't), we can take our new-found communication skills out into the field. Overconfidence leads to failure, so start small. The workplace is a major sexual minefield—it's virtually a no-fly zone for sexuality. Avoid fucking, sexualizing, or making lewd jokes around coworkers altogether. Dating co-workers is awkward and lazy. It shows folks that we probably haven't really even tried dating and implies that we'd rather talk about work than life during meals. Dating co-workers sets us up for very dull conversations but it is also potentially dangerous for our careers. Go to the field, man!

A new job is like a new relationship. Initially we feel lucky to have it. When we applied for the job, we were an enthusiastic, qualified, team-playing go-getter. At the interview we were dedicated to making sales, retaining customers, and participating in the company culture. Less than a year later, our feelings and motivations have substantially changed. At the beginning, we set the bar high and wanted to prove ourselves, but after success sank in, we became entitled. We disregarded mentorship and greedily rubbed our palms in mediocre delight.

By rejecting training programs and failing to work at our weaknesses, we slowly slip into the background. We accomplish the daily tasks, but grow insecure in our position because of change and competition. The lack of extra-curricular training makes us increasingly unreliable in moments of uncertainty. Envy creeps in and we feel that others are getting ahead of us. That high bar we set at the beginning sinks lower. We start believing our own negativity. Each time our ineptitude goes on display, we get spiteful and privately mutter insults at the competition. All the while we're angrily wondering why we are not being recognized for our contributions. We've been in this job a whole year and we show up on time every day. We don't get stoned at lunch, and we never sexually harass anyone. We nod and say, "Yes, ma'am," and, "Right away, sir" in a fashion so chipper that the competition thinks we're spineless. The competition will appear to work less and benefit more. Their contribution to the positive atmosphere is received better than our complacency. Obsolesce is right around the corner, but heart failure (or a destructive freak-out) might come first. HR would like to know ahead of time if we're feeling "duress".

This territory (of insecurity and entitlement) is ripe for angry men. Feel free to re-read the above metaphor and apply it to romantic relationships. Just know that marriage and a job are not entirely what make a man happy or healthy. If we think marriage equals sex and acceptance, and a job equals satisfaction, then we're in for some serious disappointment. We must continually work at being happy. This means adjusting to the developing needs of our sexual partners, friends, and workplaces. Obsolescence applies to work and sex. If we expect work and women to complete us, we're totally fucked. Men need to actively participate in their interests and seek opportunities for fun outside of money, intoxication, and sex.

We don't deserve everything we think we do. Even after we get what we think we want, we still aren't guaranteed happiness. Earning, striving, and being rewarded for our passion is where the gold is. Here are the steps to get out of this stratified and materialistic pickle.

Step 1: Live Smart. Don't even think about complaining, you have your solutions. Find some fucking zest, dude. You're officially in decline. If life's daily duties seem like a hassle, realize that that's just being lazy. Life is a fight against gravity, poverty, and ourselves. Gravity alone will crush the life out of us. It takes a lot of energy to live and the less we put in, the less we get out. So get down to business! There are no days off; life's work is about living it.

Step 2: Cover your basics. Sleep, water, and diet will stop your entitled mind from thinking it's better than your body. One reason you might feel unsure about life is your shitty health maintenance. You avoid hypocritical entitlement just by saying, "I need more sleep". We all need sleep, we all have financial needs. Our needs are neither bigger nor smaller than anyone else's—the challenge is articulating them clearly. Water and a semi-decent diet are no-brainers. Covering our personal health needs is important. When we feel entitled to our status more than our wellbeing, we fail to respectfully enjoy the benefit of life. It's a dick move.

Step 3: Earn and learn. Being inept is the only way to learn. All athletes begin as a puny novice. All lovers begin nervous, fumbling, and unsure. Learning athletics by watching TV is as stupid as thinking pornography will teach us how to sustain a love life. We do not make the roster without experience. We must get our hands and knees scrapped on the court to become even close to success. Same goes for work and sex. Become a landscaper. Work as a dishwasher. Go receive unprepared anal sex. What you will discover is that the learning experience can be surprisingly unpleasant. But at least you'll have learned something. Education might be unpleasant, but it should not be given up on.

Step 4: Humble thyself. Have a fucking breakdown! We were misguided by our post-war parents who helped us believe that the world was our oyster. It isn't. We can't afford oysters, and the aphrodisiac effect is lost on our limp dicks. Weep, poor little man. Weep like an emotionally undeveloped child. We can't change the world because we can't change ourselves. Luck is all we have to thank for not being dead. A shitty job, a ragged home, and single human friend is better than most. Life's okay. That disappointment you feel is socially manufactured. Let's celebrate existence and try to compare ourselves to others less often. Give up that grandiose, egotistical self-image. It helps no one. It actually distances us from long-term supportive relationships. Become like a curious, playful boy—be humble, confidant, curious, and grateful. Then seek love and good work.

We want to be special, but we don't always feel that way, so we compensate. We try to be special to someone else. This often fails or falls short of our expectation if we're not treating ourselves kindly. What mothers and past girlfriends have told us about our specialness does not apply globally. Maybe we were special for a moment when we were recognized at work (or had sex) but that feeling clearly fades. Becoming genuinely interested in what life has to offer will help us legitimately earn praise and avoid being a hypocritical douche bag. The only thing that is special about us is the bacteria behind our teeth.

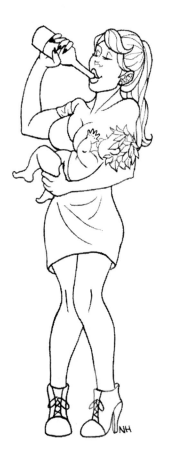

13.
Generations of Stupidity

The pinnacle of outdated manliness has been defined as a preparedness to die for what one believes in. Alternatively, to this masculine madness, children make an excellent excuse for men to keep living. If we're lucky, life can offer us babies! Raising them happy and healthy is absolutely proof of our incredible manliness. However, many of us (godless, sexless, brutish, and nerdy) men believe more in diddling ourselves than rearing babies, and that's a fucking shame. Our right to stroke our dicks while eating pre-packed burritos is not the true modern meaning of life. On the day legions of men are prepared to die for gluttony and pornography, I will admit that I was wrong. Such a blood-pact would require unpredicted devotion to hedonism, especially considering that forming a legion would require outdoor participation from shlubs. Nevertheless, if men are prepared to die for gluttony and pornography, so be it. Like the protesting monks of Chinese occupation, light yourselves on fire in protest of ejaculation control and fast food.

To the couch diddlers: is there anything worth sacrificing for? Self-serving Mom's burritos in her basement guarantees some isolation and bitterness. And babies? These men don't want babies (thank god)! Babies would necessitate social skills and having to care about something other than their dicks and stomachs. Breeding? Ha! Another one of that guy? Babies are scary for everyone when fathers can't get their shit together.

Despite civilization and obesity, men can still fuck like animals. Animals fuck to ensure the continuity of their species. Men fuck for similar reasons. Babies are men's only option for genetic continuity and that means having relations with a women. A tiny part of every man wants a baby, whether he likes himself or not. That tiny part needs monitoring, especially if he thinks the baby will:
  - Give purpose to his otherwise empty life.
  - Provide a weak person for him to treat as badly as his father treated him.
  - Make him less angry, because finally someone will love him.
  - Cause him to freak out, pretend it doesn't exist,
  run away, and deny all responsibility.
  - Allow him to run away grinning, knowing that his genes will live on.
  - Arrive accidently and leave him yelling, "How the fuck did that happen!?"
  If one of those scenarios has already occurred, you should apologize if you can.

As males, we are biologically driven to impregnate someone—being sick and poor is definitely a disadvantage. But regardless of our filth, poverty, and idiocy, most men would likely prefer to sexually succeed than not. But we're fucking ourselves up because our modern biological connection is pretty much non-existent. It has come to the point where our ignorance and ill health is literally threatening the extinction of our shlubby genetics. Non-reproduction is going to happen to many men for many reasons, so fatherhood is an extra special opportunity! Over the next generations, men will be slipping into a sterile state of sexless obesity unless there is a radical health intervention. This, however, will allow alpha males or top-notch sperm donors to rule the primordial soup for the next centuries to come.

The best of men will get the best of women, but since we're mostly uggos, our lot in life might not be as pornographic as we fantasize. The transition from post-war romance systems to pornographic fuck festivals has been… strange. Theoretically men and women are now both breadwinners—because that's awesome (or an economic necessity) for children. However, hypothetically, we have potentially doubled the workforce in the last fifty years. This has made competition naturally larger and more diverse. Reacting negatively to the change of women's role in society is really gonna hold men back in life.

A man's reactionary threats towards the advancement of women's role in society is practically proof of his non-breeding status. Dick-faced comments (online and in the streets) show a heightened desire to control women and, in a roundabout fashion, show how desperately men want women's attention (and their baby-making equipment). Life is less likely to involve reproduction for these kinds of men. It is ridiculous how men un-man themselves by blaming women rather than change themselves to accommodate them. It's pathetic and desperate to demand that the women's movement yield to men's discomfort and conformist aggression. The victims of unhealthy masculinity just need to apply physical distance and take care of themselves. The isolated males will die out from heart disease (or accident) long before they get off their masturbation station and take action on their threats. When that time comes, I'll be rocking the #1 spot at the sperm bank.

Resist becoming a sexless, pox-faced, fat-assed, dildo-loving, healthcare liability (who will die alone on a toilet from heart failure) stroking his wart-covered cock in clammy hands while letting his lonely ejaculations represent the trajectory of his embarrassing life.

Please don't breed without these tips:

Step 1: Like babies. Every day a man has a morning woody, that's his body saying yes to babies. Now obviously, if we made one baby per erection we would have an international population crisis. Enter the worthiness of masturbation and condoms. Simply like babies. Go ahead and love em'. Babies will grow up to become a significant part of our future. It takes a long time. There's no quick remedy for the kids these days. We'll just have to learn to love someone forever.

Step 2: Stink less. Our lifestyle is the problem here. Unchecked, men's habits can be terrible. Our diet, exercise pattern, and hygiene will transfer onto our children. Our toxic bullshit will poison our kids. Sometimes women can detect this toxic quality pre-sexually and weed out the unfit males. An unhealthy man will produce unhealthy children—that's a deal-breaker.

Step 3: Apply effort. Father the child regardless of divorce. Self-improvement will be required. As a lazy, underemployed douche bag, there are many reasons not to have a child—sudden change being the most accessible. So before leaping at the nearest consent-ing female to have unprotected sex, consider this: if I have acciden-tal babies how will I cope with the rapid change into fatherhood? See a doctor, get treated for shock. What society needs from fathers is incongruent with how many men are living. Be a man. Be as prepared as possible, and when in doubt, improvise.

Step 4: Commit your life. This is the end of you as a self-serving prick. Now you are Daddy. For about thirty years, expect mul-tiple personal identity crises. You will never get your reckless-self back again. But you will discover is that committing your life to something is a significant key to happiness. This can happen by accident. So smarten up the fuck up, fast, and hunker down for the long haul.

Those "*maybe* I can raise a child" guys can go fuck themselves. There is a cata-strophic lack of healthy male role models and it's our own goddamn dicks' fault. *Maybe,* pfft, you will never forgive yourself for running out on a child. Face the fears of inadequacy—you're good enough right now as you are; just man up,

Daddy-o—yes it is scary. This is your time to finally have something worth dying for.

Now, go have some loving and consensual sex. Make a baby and name it Ryan (it means little king!). All it needs is food, shelter, water, clothes, and you. It needs you, big guy.

Babies aren't complicated. Take a deep breath. You will be a new man nine months after conception.

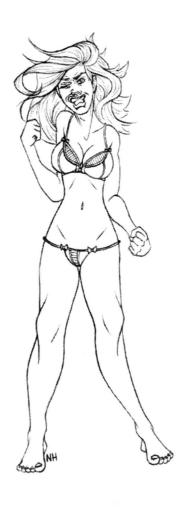

14.

Mental Health, Everyone Has It

Yup, mental health is a real thing. Everyone has it. It's good and bad. It comes and goes. Men have it but pretend they don't until they can't hide it anymore. When men experience it, it can happen unexpectedly. They can snap into awfulness or crash into misery without even knowing it happened. Every man has a couple moments he'd rather forget. In fact, he probably has a list of mistakes and flashback memories that still sting. The men who deny or ignore their own mental health get screwed out of honest relationships and the consequences can be deadly. Addictions and stupid habits just cover up men's crazy bullshit. A man can cover up his bullshit for the rest of his life alone, or he can face the pain by seeking support in his daily life.

Somewhere inside our minds, we've got traumas. They need resolution because they create shitty mental blocks, bad patterns, and negative expectations. In turn these can fuck up our relationship with ourselves and others. If we haven't realized the influence of our childhoods or never meaningfully connected with anyone, how can we get advice when nobody really knows us? Somewhere there is a list of common traumas that men experience, and I'd wager most of us have one—injury and embarrassments being most common.

I would bet that most folks have experienced (or perceive) some form of trauma in their lives. Everybody has pain, and pain has a source. I would also bet that, as a man, we've never actively sought emotional support outside of our sex lives—if that. I don't mean professional help necessarily, I mean explicitly asking friends to listen and support us in hard times. Most men, I fear, let past trauma penetrate their essential character by numbing it alone. Men's internal monologues of isolation, aggression and regret vary wildly but they all will manifest in some form of addiction, disease, or rage.

Instead of admitting that we are all a little bit messed up right now, many men choose to self-medicate. But this is inherently isolating. Pot smokers get together and date other pot smokers, and they never have zest again. Drunks get drunk with other drunks and scream until they start to cry. Crack smokers, cocaine users, heroin addicts, and meth folks are all numbing themselves with like-minded company. What is that? It's a lack of connection in the community.

Recovery begins when we start to listen to our thoughts kindly. In the darkest times, kindness is most needed and furthest away. That nagging voice gets louder as we approach deeper misery. More misery demands more self-medication. The nagging voice tells us to smarten up, drink less, sleep more, and eat better. But the hangover says, "Eat crap, water, water, whiskey, water. Maybe if that girl will cuddle me, I'll feel better. Nope, cuddles don't fix shit, whiskey, whiskey…" Loneliness, exhaustion, and hangovers make us feel like a waste of space. Bam, now we've got lethargic sadness. Now we're having another drink or six to solve this hangover depression. Then after four or six hangovers in a row, our bodies start to slow way down. We start thinking, "I'm slow, I'm stupid, and I'm hopeless. Maybe if I go to the bar, maybe if I beat this game, maybe if a girl will sleep with me, I'll feel better." The next morning she leaves because we've neglected to buy groceries and we've got no breakfast plan. The cycle is reinforced the next weekend when our buddies (who also drink like idiots) come over to drink, yell, bromance, and laugh until women don't matter. Then we all puke and pass out, never questioning anything. Recovery starts the moment we start contemplating the patterns we don't want anymore.

Don't know where to go? Who do you talk to about this? Do all your friends keep getting you drunk? Are you still having fun? Why are you so frequently unhappy and angry? Are you self-medicating? Do you have supportive friends? Do you try so hard to fit in that being yourself is a bad thing?

Mental health, dear friend, it's called mental health

Somewhere inside of every douche bag is a happy little boy. At some point (very early on), that little boy, well, he got screwed up and became you. If you can identify those moments of change and face them, sober and calm, this might encourage a woman to stick around and be patient with you.

Some steps.

> Step 1: Trauma. At some point every man has had his childhood destroyed forever (ie: Santa is not real, puppies die, head injury, or sexual molestation). On top of that, we fuck it up worse with negative responses and by ignoring our problems (aka: walking it off). In this state of emotional repression, we unknowingly inflict collateral damage by being guarded or defensive or in denial about our mental health and that pushes supporters away. The sooner we can recover from this stuff and stop sugar-coating life with insecurity or bravado, the healthier we'll be.

> Step 2: Don't fix this alone. Lonely men lack perspective, but still have arms that need an occupation. Frankly, a lot of a guy's friends serve little purpose beyond keeping them sane. A mental-health recovery might require actually going out into the community and

participating in activities outside of our comfort zones. It is possible to recover but isolation breeds stagnation and addiction makes for toxic friend circles. Support is needed and effort is required.

Step 3: Fuck toxic relationships. As stated earlier, many of our friends suck. Our collective masculine identity is unnecessarily ugly, manufactured, and unfriendly. Keeping toxic friends significantly impacts our ability to change. Keeping shitty friends is a reflection on us. Get out of toxic groups before your only sexual option becomes prostitutes and dudes who can keep a secret. I'm still developing a term for "a man whose female sexual options are so few that he has no other choice than to secretly engage in gay sex—despite the fact that he isn't really attracted to men and feels shame for it." Backscratcher is the going term. Backscratchers include (but are not limited to) drunks, the steroid using, the drug addled, the uggos, the lonely, and the pornography addicted. Ditch unsupportive friends and go find new ones.

Step 4: Change. Oh man, facing personal pain will definitely be less enjoyable than masturbating. It is totally an option to ignore our emotional bullshit forever. Though unpleasant and scary, the cure lies in kindness. Men who are gentler with themselves will get more happiness and sex at the cost of temporary emotional discomfort. But wait, happiness and sex are always temporary! Men who reach a comfortable mediocrity and let their balls wither won't win in the long run either. It's us healthy dudes, rocking-out with the life-time self-improvement, who will keep getting invited back to the pussy party.

As the troglodytes of the Great Man Caves say: "Epic fail, bro." Men need this book more than their hopeless fantasies of one day being sexually dominant. We have mental health problems simply by having no realistic purpose for our penis.

Go on, be brave. Ask for some help. The sooner the better. Emotions aren't life-threatening.

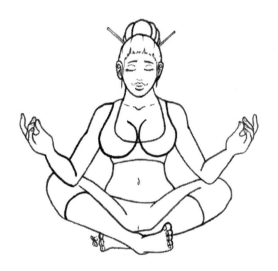

15.

Feeling Feelings. Many Suck

In this section, I'll be using some words that you might never have heard before. Instead of the standard steps to fix your shit, I've made a list of feelings. In the future when you are feeling feelings and aren't sure what that means, this list might help. Add your own! Underline the useful ones!

There are two culturally acceptable man-feelings that men swing back-and-forth from: aggression (angry) and elation (happy). Feelings are much more plentiful than this; however, these ones receive the most social permission from our male peers. When situations arise and force men to feel more complex feelings, this becomes problematic due to our crappy emotional vocabulary. Without basic emotional competency, men easily become mentally exhausted by vacillating between complex unknown emotions. This will naturally lead to his agitation. One way or another, his complex feeling will erupt. Our spouse, girlfriend, divorce lawyer, parole officer, even our grandma will be able to draw out complex feelings. An emotionally stupid man will feel as if they are punishing him by forcing him to feel feelings. Belligerently, he'll state, "I don't want to talk about it!" What that means is that nobody gets to understand what the fuck is going on with him. The only thing we are aware of is his rising blood pressure, body language, and tone of voice—he looks angry and dangerous.

What we express is a reflection of what we are feeling. Anger disguises complex feelings and generally amplifies our problems. Unfortunately, too often anger is personified as distinctly masculine. Thus, men practice this emotion most. Anger is effective; it deflects other even more unpleasant feelings. This benefits us because we can avoid change and appear strong. Unfortunately anger leaves us abandoned, repeatedly, which reinforces our emotional isolation. Anger is the de-facto go-to emotion for hiding complex repressed man-feelings. But it's a trap! Remember shouting, "I'm not angry. I just don't want to talk about it." Well, mister smarty pants, what *are* you feeling then?

The second fundamental man-feeling is happiness. Artificial happiness happens after two drinks, but it vanishes after five. We might not even remember the last time we felt truly happy. Sometimes we mistake feeling F.I.N.E. for feeling happy. It is a common confusion. To be truly happy, we require the complete fulfillment of all our needs—seriously. Food, shelter, water, and clothing are fundamental needs that our world must accommodate if we are ever going to have safe communities. However, in North American we are conditioned to live beyond our basic needs and that makes us addicted and perpetually unsatisfied. Rent drives us crazy. Love drives us crazy. Binge drinking drives us crazy. The whole system can drive us crazy. When lonely folks see happy couples, it creates a false sense of worthlessness. It can be very difficult to actually be happy.

Doubts sucks, but our escape from despair is the pursuit of happiness. Happiness is the rebellion against fear, it is a great feeling! There are many reasons to be fearful: debt, underemployment, fatness, isolation, cost of living, war, technology, and much more. But when we have food, shelter, water and clothing, why aren't we happy?

Believe it or not, many of us are happy but get fucked over because we want so much more out of life. Men must recognize that multiple emotions can be felt at the same time. Happiness can exist during a period of unfulfilled ambition. We feel anger and happiness simultaneously when we put on a fake smile for someone we dislike. Whether we know it or not, unknown feelings (which you will learn to articulate below) are turning us into emotional rollercoasters and total assholes. Expressing complex feelings requires practice. It's uncomfortable but it is not life threatening. We don't need to know everything right away, but if we stay in this state of emotional confusion, we risk becoming frigid, numb, and rejected. In turn, that will ruin our sex lives and make our social groups unsupportive. Raw happiness is impossibly idealistic and though it is easily synthesized with drugs and alcohol, it comes down to short-sighted emotional avoidance. Yes, there are many feelings that we would rather not feel. Well tough shit. Eventually something will permanently change our lives without permission. Identifying complex feelings will make us more graceful during this crisis. It is very easy to ignore our feelings and needs; the problem lies in our eruptions and degenerating health. Don't be that guy.

Man's emotional vocabulary desperately needs improvement. Unless he has studied psychology or been through therapy, the emotions listed will be new. This is nobody's fault; it's just the result of an archaic educational system that won't validate man's preference for vulgarity.

Glossary of Sucky Feelings: I feel _____

Rage	Self-righteous	Suffering	Drained	Guarded
Attacked	Lonely	Stupid	Disrespected	Unsatisfied
Anxious	Unavailable	Grumpy	Hypoglycemic	Untrustworthy
Desperate	Suicidal	Escape	Purposeless	Delusional
Touchy	Abandoned	Panic	Skeptical	Afraid
Anger	Self-important	Pain	Pitiful	Overwhelmed
Defensive	Rejected	Explosive	Flawed	Scattered
Emasculated	Unsure	Disconnected	Impatient	Berserk
Uninspired	Estranged	Unloved	Spiteful	Breakdown
Cocky	Catastrophizing	Mediocre	Suspicious	Troubled
Frustrated	Egotistical	Ignorant	Pathetic	Burnt out
Hostile	Shameful	Derogatory	Incurable	Skittish
Violent	Restless	Insignificant	Worried	Manic
Stuck	Unfamiliar	Disapproving	Dangerous	Murderous
Stern	Yearning	Lazy	Resentful	Disturbed
Doubt	Hurt	Useless	Reckless	Annoyed
Regretful	Embarrassed	Stagnant	Boring	Shy
Hateful	Reclusive	Hopeless	Possessive	Careless
Ugly	Questioning	Confused	Singled out	Fake
Unforgiving	Obsessive	Lethargic	Unready	Volatile
Troubled	Blaming	Unheard	Needy	Depressed
Apologetic	Wanting	Fussy	Unsafe	Nervous
Numb	Disgusted	Helpless	Denial	Remorse
Dread	Lust	Jealous	Directionless	Agitated

Glossary of Happy Feelings: I feel _____

Fit	Expectant	Prepared	Easygoing	Truthful
Present	Hopeful	Engaged	Elated	Understood
Joy	Stylish	Aroused	Euphoric	Confident
Thrilled	Proud	Achievement	Fulfilled	Intelligent
Orgasmic	Unique	Tickled	Full	Worthy
Thoughtful	Loved	Focused	Genuine	Honoured
Elation	Supported	Amused	Glad	Capable
Kind	Heard	Charitable	Golden	Open
Philosophic	Satisfied	Agreeable	Groovy	Determined
Philanthropic	Special	Amazed	Honest	Studious
Validated	Humble	Amazing	Joyful	Assured
Generous	Professional	Blessed	Jubilant	Surprised
In Control	Motivated	Blissful	Funny	Righteous
Glad	Relaxed	Bright	Praiseworthy	Certain
Respected	Inspired	Certain	Prosperous	Levity
Inventive	Included	Cheerful	Real	Committed
Connected	Ready	Childlike	Reliable	Gravity
Creative	Organized	Clear	Romantic	Keen
Respectful	Pleased	Committed	Safe	Faithful
Fabulous	Welcoming	Skillful	Secure	Pleasant
Sexy	Chillin'	Confident	Sincere	Stimulated
Well	Fired-up	Content	Careful	Accountable
Dressed	Stoked	Contented	Sensitive	Available
Enticed	Comfortable	Distracted	Stoked	Supportive
Intrigued	Clean	Dreamy	Thoughtful	In-need

Book 2
The Advanced Chapters

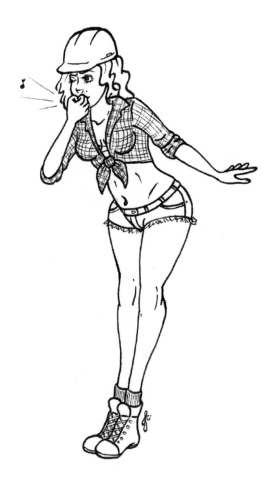

16.
Watching the girls go by? Try smiling!

Eye contact and a smile is the best possible outcome when crossing paths with an unknown woman. Men who gawk at women on the streets tend to observe their age, tits, legs, ass, neckline, style, and then face—in that order. Since before stretchy pants hit the market, men have veered many cars into lampposts while rubber-necking like Albertan tourists in Times Square. This rubber-necking at chicks is hopeless and shows how unfamiliar men are face-to-face with ladies.

Because we suck in conversations with women, bikinis (and the other shiny things women wear) present great opportunities for curbside stupidity relapse and fender-benders. Gawking at women while driving is only slightly less dangerous than text-messaging and driving, making these men a legitimate threat to public safety. This gape response is made substantially worse by cat calling because it makes the threat known. Hollering at women in the streets identifies a man as an insecure douche bag. This compulsive eye-fucking and cat-calling becomes group behaviour when it is reinforced by our buddies through passive agreement. Groups of douche bags are easily identified and quickly avoided by women. Also they make poor quality friends. When men start bitching about women in general, it's obvious they don't know very many of them. Most women are smart, funny, and kind, and they have a low tolerance for bullshit.

When we lose our train of thought upon the sight of a human female and begin a "hey buddy look at that one" shtick, it reinforces our group's isolation from women. These guys act like poorly trained dogs who would charge a bitch if it wasn't for civilization. If that is your group's shtick, none of you are worthy of the things you want and, individually, your push-over conformity to toxic masculinity is a fucking joke.

At a distance, our eyes fixate on her hips and tits, but we'd sniff her crotch if we could. However, we can't. She won't let us. We don't even know this person. Cat-calling is the response for idiots without realistic sexual communication skills. We might spot a woman from a balcony or from behind a work fence, or while we're driving, and suddenly feel compelled to holler "you a sexy bitch baby" (or something to that effect) before running off to inform our buddies about some local eye-candy. Stop. Don't. We'll be better off. Both choices (showing your buddies a hottie and hollering at her) lead to aggressive patterns towards women that will drive healthy sex out of our lives.

The deeply incompetent men out there have excuses to avoid women like, "She's probably a slut." But what he really says is, "I'm probably not good enough for her." Sadly, that's much more accurate however it is, at least, an actionable personal improvement opportunity. She might have a spectacular sex life! Jealous? On the other hand, she might have learned that "all" men are baboons and opt not to have a sex life. Through negative learning environments, some women have come to learn that men are altogether avoidable. When men wear stupid like a badge of honor, they become sexually unapproachable.

Maybe we holler at a woman from across the street, or perhaps we just share comments with buddies. Either way we get further from actually talking to a real woman. When we happen to pass by a youthful human female, check her tits, and then sharply look away, we reveal a lack of integrity in our intention— and sunglasses. It is uncomfortable being called out for ogling. We solve this problem simply by looking people in the eyes and smiling. That's it, that's all! Yer' done! She won't stop and suddenly want to love-fuck. A woman resists making eye contact with men because she fears that she'll accidently send a positive message and he will start following her around. Men's longstanding possessiveness and neediness is super fucking destructive. Our lack of basic emotional confidence keeps us trapped in our man-caves forever. Just politely smile at women and move along. Just notice people respectfully. That is way sexier.

Looking is very different than ogling, then hollering, and then saying raunchy things about her to our buddies. Hollering is rude and it makes people feel vulnerable. It shows we lack class and clearly don't deserve a conversation. When we drool, smack our lips, and talk about the contours of her clothing, we consolidate our sexual shallowness as a fundamental value in our male peer group. Any relationship these types of men enter will possess doubts of fidelity and increase the likelihoods of angry divorce.

Are you dating hoes? If she is a hoe, then you are dirt. I am the fucking fertilizer. I'm giving you the shit you need to grow bigger. That's a metaphor, dick. Advance your ability to use language respectfully (and maybe even eloquently) and women (perhaps even yourself) will find you intelligent. Words like hoe, bitch, cunt, tramp, slut, whore, and whatever trash your rat brain came up with should be scrapped permanently. You will be lucky if your girlfriend is even slightly more attractive than you. You are not a ten, okay? You won't ever fuck a ten, like the ones in porn and the movies. Tens work in specialized industries with security budgets for a reason. It takes effort like makeup, a wardrobe, self-confidence, and mental health maintenance to be a famous porn star or celebrity babe. You ain't got a fifth of that hustle. So don't pretend, and don't let your loud mouth get your balls in trouble.

Here are some charm tips for the varying degrees of female-contact that you might experience:

Step 1: Smile, no contact. When you encounter the human female, a rush of blood might surge into your penis. You might mistake this for love. It isn't. Continue what you are doing. I know you really want that woman to notice you, but do not act out. Smile and look bashful. That is a more accurate representation of what you are currently feeling. Being genuine will get easier with practice. If she is across the street, try an outward smile and an internal sigh. Again, it is a more realistic representation of what you are feeling. If you are rowdy and hollering, by the time you get your smile out, she'll already be scared off.

Step 2: Smile, passing contact. This time, don't turn your head or miss your stride, but smile at her face. When you accidently stumble, it is a sign of nervousness and can be very cute. Be subtle and brief in your eye contact and smile. If all you're doing is smiling, you don't need to be afraid of her noticing that you're looking. When you hold back your jackass comments and resist the impulse to intimidate women, then the real, fallible you is showing. If there is a connection, like she smiles back, your heart might begin to flutter slightly. Many men take this as a cue to flex or say something stupid. Just say hello and move on; this is practicing respect.

Step 3: Smile, momentary contact. At some point, you might actually have a brief conversation with a human female. Perhaps the grocery clerk or the banker. If you are intent on engaging in flirtation but you aren't good with women, say so. Smile and say something nice. You don't have to buy shots, make jokes, or tell some embellished story. Just smile and say something positive. Or tell her some good news, or something that happened recently. Follow it up with what you've learned from it. Ask her if she has had any good news lately, listen, and then tell her that it was nice to meet her. Done.

Step 4: Smile, prolonged contact. If you have somehow convinced a woman to spend an extended period with you (aka: a date), don't screw it up by being a shit head. Don't use tricks or dismantle her self-confidence with backhanded compliments. The more honest you are from the start, the better. Share in the conversation as equally as possible. Accomplishments, friends, and activities are awesome topics of conversation, but not as interesting as ideas, feelings, and dreams. So smile and talk about the man you are and who you hope to become. (Pro tip: ask questions about her interests.)

The embellishment of men's sexual conquests is a sad joke; it is a painfully competitive homo-social-sexual pissing match that makes outsiders cringe. Everyone just wants someone to accept them. Bravado serves to get validation from other stupid lonely men, but not women. Why are we so full of shit with our friends and such jackasses to women?

When asking a woman out for a date you get one and a half attempts. If and when you have a woman's attention, don't go over the top. Desperation and fear of loneliness is why we react so strongly to rejection and cling on to toxic man-friends. Quit hiding.

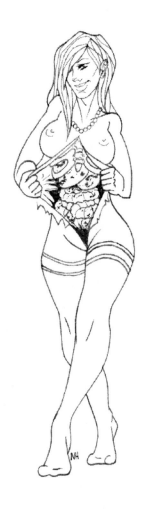

17.

Ugly on the Inside

Delusional lust can never be reasonably attained and it will erode our attachment to reality. Though some attractive women have said, "I'm not really into looks," they are still seeking someone intelligent, inspired, and amazing. Tens occasionally date down, and boy, is that good news for our delusions. But it's irrelevant because that would necessitate inspiration and motivation. Most folks are average (Fives); they should be realistic with how far they intend to date up—anything outside of a reasonable +1 is delusional lust without some good talent backing it up. If a man is truly a unicorn (a man who fucks women who are massively more attractive than himself), he's probably a fan-fucking-tastic all around guy.

Men, we are not unicorns, and conversations about tits are not the key to dating up. No incredibly capable woman deeply craves ass compliments. Don't mistake her uncomfortable giggle with a cue to follow up. When our necks bend for every pair of yoga pants and every set of cleavage, our internal ugly is showing.

When we obsess about artificial physical beauty, local beauty loses its lustre. We become critical of ourselves and appear condescending of imperfection. This manufactured expectation will become so unrealistic that the women who meet our standard will be virtually non-existent. Dissatisfaction with women reflects dissatisfaction of the self. Believing too much in the myth of physical beauty will lead to serious disappointments when we're old.

If we are intent on dating a world-class woman, become deserving of it. We suck at cooking, are terrible at cleaning, and we were never trained to maintain a garden or raise a child. It takes a lot of cash to keep up good appearances but it takes a lot of effort to maintain one's health and relationships. Men need to put some investment into their personal appearance and simultaneously care about themselves inwardly. Personal maintenance prevents us rotting from the inside out. We are all complex emotional creatures. Expecting pornographic sex, unconditional love, and an infinitely high tolerance for our bullshit is too much to ask from a spouse. We might have a decent face and be rotten on the inside, or we might be terribly ugly and deeply inspired. It may not feel fair, and to make it worse, we all get uglier and stupider as we get old. It's unavoidable. It's gravity and obsolescence. And it's the nature of generational social recalibrating. Every man must mind his health today, in order to maintain his dick and dignity later in life.

Have you got any health prevention strategies in place? Do you eat vegetables? Are your shits like shards of plastic? Have you gone to the dentist lately, or seen a doctor? Being dependent on female-relationship caregiving will lead you into a total health crapshoot.

Here are some tips, but you ain't gonna like them:

Step 1: Get fit. Muscular atrophy makes a man particularly ugly on the inside and outside. A lazy lifestyle will infect our relationships and lead to a brief life and heart troubles. Quality of life declines substantially with respiratory difficulty, cardiovascular weakness, mobility struggles, and the associated mental health decline. At a certain point of fatness and poor circulation it will become a struggle to identify penis/vagina contact. The decay of our physical body will compound our mental health problems and solidify negative thought patterns. Getting fit is one way to break these patterns. Begin training for something, anything. Fitness is one way to be kind to our bodies and stave off the inside uglies.

Step 2: Eat right. A healthy diet is experiential and is taught over a lifetime. The $1.25 sandwich fits into our budget and our rapid-fire lifestyle. The flat of beer fits into our budget and our social life. But the financial commitment to fruit and vegetables doesn't make the cut? The crappy quality of food and beverage turns our insides ugly. Symptoms like anal fissures and lethargy are the body telling us we're feeling nasty. Gut pain is not just hunger but an unhappy body trying to tell us something. We're addicted to crappy food.

Step 3: Daily work. Be realistic with exercises and do them every day! Life takes place every single day after each night's sleep. Exercise becomes fun once we hit our stride and aren't in pain, so take it slow. Everyone has tried exercising before and failed to keep it up. Are we just fucking giving up forever? Get out and fucking do it! Every fucking day! Don't bank on erections after thirty if you are fucking your life up in your twenties.

Step 4: Lower the bar. The best way for us to meet the bar is to lower it. Don't worry about becoming *Mr. Men's Health*—that magazine is just as shameful as *Cosmo*—just be happy with who you are becoming. Pace yourself, don't be perfectionists. There are very few opinions that matter in life. Make yours one of them. If you can't meet other people's expectations, fuck them. But remember that we do want to live up to some of them. Stop looking outwards and turn in to seek your satisfaction—this will draw in the right people.

We don't ever see a top athlete sex-bomb married to an angry and obese man.

Put effort in for the rest of your life. Comparing a real human woman to an internet woman will only push real relationships further away. Only once our egos and expectations have become realistic and articulated will we feel successful. Unrealistic fantasies can make partners feel ugly and inadequate. That's not fair.

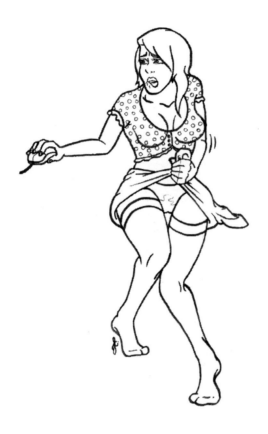

18.
Pornography, a Lifestyle

I am pleased to announce the official existence of pornography as an all-new. The pornophile! Everyone will be thrilled to discover how satisfying the pornography lifestyle can truly be. It comes with no danger from actually encountering other humans! The average male no longer needs to feel fear of rejection, abandonment, insecurity, or obsolescence. Sex is always on hand! This sexual preference can suit even the most delusional of males. Plus, there is no risk of sexually transmitted infection or pregnancy. To accommodate, permit, and even inspire our perpetual sexual isolation, the sex industry has gladly produced vagina-like (and anus-like) tools for our penises to slip into instead.

Never again will we have to swallow pubic hair in our righteous quest for a squirt to the face. Nor will we ever have to taste the sweat of another person. No bodily fluids will ever be exchanged, and we can finally achieve our lifelong dream of sexual sanitation, perversion, and ejaculation freedom. Save money on dates, condoms, and shared meals. Don't forget to stock up on lubricant and buy yourself a stroker! Just squint and imagine fucking anyone and anything, anytime you want!

Be it throat fucking, gangbanging, cuckoldry, or fucking machines, now we can imagine ourselves as any type of sexual hero through the magic of the internet. For the low price of an internet hook up and a basic computer, we can all jack ourselves to unrestricted sexual bliss forever.

For adventurous men, I recommend ass dildos. The internet can provide a great amount of sexual satisfaction, but so can an ass dildo! Why waste time trying to talk with women when we can just go fuck ourselves? Dabble in emotionally risk-free conversations with women in the online chat rooms. Men can get hours of unresponsive pleasure from sending sexual messages to (theoretically) real "women" online. We can describe our wildest fantasies and attach photographs of our semi-erect dicks. Be sure to have a credit card ready!

Be warned, sometimes we can get deleted from dating sites for making lewd comments and threats. Just make a new account with fake pictures! Remember, each sexually harassing message must be unique to outwit the troll-bots. When we write, "Sit on my face and call my Sally!" we have to type it out every time.

Fortunately, there are hundreds of sites that offer free memberships exclusively to men because they are overflowing with pussy. All of them host thousands of women who are waiting to fuck you. Yes, you! I know, right? And you can have sex with everyone, every night! You'll never be lonely again. Thanks to the mysteries of the internet, BBWs, grannies galore, imported brides, and lonely housewives all want to fuck you now.

Every woman on the internet craves one-night stands with pale, limp-dicked, agoraphobic men. Don't ejaculate until you see what you paid for! Otherwise, you might lose interest and go back to video gaming or Netflix.

If a man ejaculates too quickly, there is information available on pornography sites for that too. Online resources are available to grow a bigger dick, discover the elusive female orgasm, and create a pornography network and virtual harem—all from the comfort of our masturbation stations. At last, every man can add any woman who has ever videotaped herself naked to his favorites list. To make these great offers even more fabulous, they have an entire call centre dedicated to responding to our messages! Who needs friends or therapists when our online chat-room attendants will literally take their clothes off while offering basic counselling services? Also, they will fuck themselves while we jerk off.

No, the webcam titty counsellors don't have to watch us masturbate. There are too many men in the chat room, but that sure makes her time valuable! Every whackadoodle can pay her for extra attention by live auction (Ladies, this might even pay more than psychiatry!). So go ahead and ask that webcam titty counsellor those difficult questions we're otherwise too afraid to ask in real life.

The downside of the pornography lifestyle is that sexual familiarity will never develop. Pornography lacks the necessary intimacy for sexual relationships in real life. Pornophiles ignore all the personality and the emotional challenge of sex. Pornophiles are inherently isolated. Their sexual expectations of women are grossly inflated. How they perform in bed will never be as good as they imagine. Over time, their sense of beauty becomes defined as a physical matter, and that will be ironic because they're incredibly ugly. With so few opportunities to interact with women, they'll be inclined towards possessiveness and drive away long lasting connections.

To a lesser extent, the pornophile within a relationship might start getting intrusive images of porn during sex or intimacy. When he finds himself up late downloading porn and masturbating while his wife is asleep half-naked, then his sexual relationship is doubtfully healthy. His masturbatory death grip will cause his penis to stop responding to soft vaginas—enter limpdick. Romance and quality time is lost. Intimacy is less stimulating because there are fewer orgasms per hour—fact. Having never had any counselling, he will mistake his behaviour as normal and not detrimental to his health and social skills whatsoever.

His sexual ineptitude will be compounded with delusional envy of porn. He will blame his significant other because she doesn't reach the gold standard of pornographic cock sucking.

We will never be the pornography hero that we imagine ourselves. Here are some tips:

Step 1: Imagination. One way to tell if our sexual orientation has become pornographic is through masturbation. Can you achieve ejaculation without pornography? Try whacking off while in bed in the dark. If you find your imaginations are unsuccessful at arousing an erection, you are a pornophile.

Step 2: Slow down. Try again, but this time with some personal intimacy. Don't start with whack-whack-whack-whack-whack-whack-whack. Really stroke that cock long and slow. Add lube, light candles, tickle your balls, stimulate your ass, squeeze your nipples, and anything else you like. Maybe you like the sexy music? This is more like actual sex. Sex takes a lot more time than clicking a video and five minutes of furious wanking. Fuck yourself in the actual environment in which you might eventually fuck someone (your bed). Familiarity will improve future performance.

Step 3: Doing without. This chronic pornography habit is leading us down a path of unfamiliarity of the emotional and physical aspects of sex. Plus, we risk erectile troubles from the masturbatory death grip. This is a masculine catastrophe! We've traded our vitality and genetic continuum for ten thousand ejaculations into the laundry! It's time to reconsider porn consumption and put the parental locks on the internet.

Step 4: Jane Austin. To understand women and be less of a pervert, I suggest men read books and watch movies written or directed by women and about women. What we will discover is that few women are pornophiles, but still have incredible sex fantasies in their imaginations. Women are put off by the over-consumption of porn. To engage in more real human contact, men, let's curb our enthusiasm for porn, learn about women's fantasies, and channel our sexual energy into something more profound than tissues.

Whacking off six times a day will leave your balls empty and your dick unresponsive. We all know the diminishing satisfaction from second, third, fourth, fifth, and sixth ejaculations, so save yourself from this void of loneliness and treat your dick with more respect.

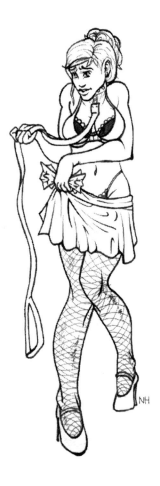

19.

For the Love of Hookers

I once met a man who told me that the majority of his sexual encounters were paid for. He was twice-married and could afford a lot of hookers. His high financial status sufficiently blinded him and his wife to his sexual stupidity. I wondered how she coped with that.

The inability to have meaningful sexual relationships will lead a man to seek sex for cash. If he wasn't so fucking ignorant, he could help himself to recover some self-esteem, but that's doubtful. Sex-workers aren't here to help us, jackass. They are here to make money from lonely men who are afraid of change. Sex-workers don't care if Johns drink too much, snort blow, shit the bed, or cry about their girlfriends. They are professional customer service providers. A good sex-trade worker will permit any stupidity up to the point where it jeopardizes her safety. All our delusions and our misguided emotions serve only to create her market demand.

Granted, there is an unlimited spectrum of sex-workers just like there is an unlimited spectrum of men who purchase their services. The men range from sexless vagrants to hooker-dependant upper class dicks. Though physically clean, the upper class dick purchases sex for scandalous reasons, whereas the sexless vagrant purchases sex as a sad novelty. Both cases present a troubling state of sexual existence; however, the sexless vagrant is (by virtue of his sadness) in far less denial than the other. Either way, the state of these men's emotional health is damaged, and too far gone to fix with casual advice—seek a professional. Johns are all emotionally volatile and develop aggressive/defensive tendencies when they are challenged. They are known for numbing their feelings and avoiding responsibility.

Is it any wonder that these women, the sex-trade workers, are the most vulnerable to violence and murder? These women are savagely abused because the men who employ their services are emotionally fucked up. These dudes need the kind of support only a mother or a whole community support network can provide. When a John discovers that Roxanne can't be mommy, he can get very upset. Sex-trade workers are never a substitute for supportive relationships! Men who purchase sex are perpetuating modern slavery. If a man is hooker-dependant, there is a litany of emotional questions that accompany that behavior. With no ability to address or understand his core problems, these men will continue to come up short.

When the thirty minutes of paid-for sex is over, those briefly forgotten feelings all return. Abandonment, rejection, inferiority, loneliness, dependence, shame, and self-loathing are not solved with sex. Being inside a woman doesn't change anything about our current rut. The prenatal security of being lovingly cuddled in a womb is not an available service from a sex worker. So we get angry with sex worker because we can't find love? No one will ever care for us like mommy. She definitely won't. She's a professional with another appointment in an hour, and she needs a wash up and reset her makeup, hair, and outfit before leaving.

Being rejected by a sex worker is inevitable. Paid-for sex involves all of the same feelings of powerlessness and inferiority of being dumped (from a real romantic relationship), but this rejection we have to pay for. The same person, the prostitute, who we don't feel should have any power over us, does. How do we reclaim that power? That's right, violence. Those fucking simpletons. A prostitute is like a cook. If we send the food back with a nasty complaint, we'll get spit in our sandwich. Men who assault a pleasure-providing prostitute should expect to get pepper sprayed, tracked down, arrested, exposed, charged, and finally prison-fucked. This might constitute reasonable justice for the victim; however, vengeance is a frightening motif and may include more extreme measures—see Medean Crisis. When released from prison, the men who honourably release the past can accept help might become emotionally articulate.

Instead of sex workers, try dating. It takes more time, emotional investment, and some disappointing rejection. This is never directly cash for sex but sometimes involves mutual expenses. Dating is the only way to meet compatible mates. Yes, it is tricky; it takes a consideration, wit, and energy to woo a woman, but have you forgotten how to flirt?

Don't worry, solutions are as follows:

Step 1: Romance. You can't romance a hooker. If you find you are spending additional cash on your favorite prostitute, then you have successfully been upsold. This imaginary emotional intimacy you share with your prostitute will not accumulate into a freebie. To be romantic, you must be beyond paying for sex. Romance is an investment in memories that make up the foundation of a relationship. That romance clarifies loving moments within a relationship.

Step 2: Get tested. Seriously, if you've been having dangerous sex, get tested for STIs and other sexually related illnesses. Get tested often and wear a lot of condoms. We're supposed to get tested after every new partner. The penis spreads diseases just as well as vaginas, but oddly sexual health clinics are packed mostly with women.

Step 3: Be alone. It takes practice being comfortable alone with your thoughts. Sexual dependence is indicative of low self-esteem, lack of an exercise routine, and a life without meaning. By using distractions like sex, games, and drugs too often, you illustrate how uncomfortable you are with your own thoughts.

Step 4: Flowers. You don't need to buy sex workers flowers; this is a misplaced romantic sentiment. Buy flowers for yourself, Cupcake. Clip the stems every two days at 45 degrees and put a bit of white sugar in the water to keep them perky. When you go on a date, cut off a single (cheesy and romantic) bloom and bring it along with you. Put it in a cup of water when you arrive at your date. This tiny romantic gesture will solidify a lasting memory for both of you— even if the date flops. It is a symbol that you are trying, and that you are not afraid to be seen as goofy and sentimental.

All right, your mom ain't coming back to take care of you. You are no longer ten. A prostitute can pretend to be your mom for a short while, but when your time is up, you're still the same repressed loser that you were before.

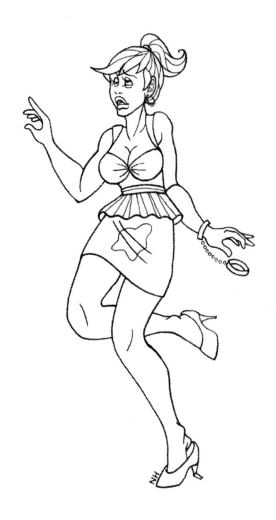

20.
You're a Drunk! Ya Drunk

When we get black-out drunk, our inner demon surfaces—and by that I mean we get wildly emotional. When we get that drunk, everyone nearby gets the pleasure of experiencing our crippled psyche. Whenever the liquor wears off (which assumes we aren't immediately re-toxifying) a sad nattering voice surfaces inside us begging for change. Phrases like "gaahh, I'm never drinking again" "ooh, fuck, I'm so sick" and "what the hell happened" can swirl into a dislikeable inner monologue. Self-pity is a sign that we feel we did something that we shouldn't have. Yes, we've poisoned ourselves and possibly damaged our reputations. At this point, this is no longer just a neutral hangover, this is an emotional hangover. We may selectively forget our behaviour but someone remembers, for sure. When we wake up feeling a sneaky suspicion that we've fucked up big time, we were probably a terrible drunk the night before. Here are a few themes of men binge-drinking:

> Peeing: Drunken men piss, sometimes on friends. They pee any-where they damn well please, including off balconies, out windows, and into city plant pots. We pee in bedroom corners at four in the morning while exhausted girlfriends stand in shock, screaming. We dress up in costumes, like vampires or queens, and piss while we rush to take down our pants. We pee in cups, jars, and buckets when we're too drunk to care. Alleyways and by-streets are marked heavily with our piss. We piss the bed sometimes when blacked-out and, when we pass-out midstream, we'll fall asleep in our piss. All of these instances can lead to arrest, lost reputation, and peeing in that tiny metal urinal in the corner of the drunk tank.

> Yelling: Many folks yell when they get drunk. It scares the shit out of friends, strangers, and lovers. When frightened, people tend to run away—women included. Drunken arguments are especially dangerous inside intimate relationships. The folks we love will leave so fast that we won't have time to get our balance before they are out the door. Saying goodbye shouldn't need screaming. Yelling at a woman who is behind a locked door will keep it locked forever. Shouting at another man is the best way to get a broken nose and non-sports related concussion. Drunken bravado is a bluff that is easy to call (anticipate a right hook). Drunks often lose, especially against cars. Yelling invites a lot of negative attention and opens a

man up to harsh situational consequences. Close calls, failure to arrest, and near-misses abound in the world of drunken bravado. Learn from other men's mistakes (watch drunken fail videos) and stop this kind of domestic violence by curbing male stupidity. Once we get seriously fucked up by the consequences, that'll really bring the point home. Learning through repercussions is a shitty way to educate ourselves.

Crying: All our anger is for nothing, and mostly it only hurts us. With a broken nose and a no relationship, sometimes men find themselves sobbing, lonely, and wasted. We drink too much when we want to feel happy but feel helpless to find happiness. Because of one's basic lack of happiness, and the abysmal void of happiness that results from excessive drinking, we realize there is no happiness at the end of this strategy. There is no force of nature that can change the course of our lives other than ourselves, and right now we can barely walk. In a drunken stupor we clearly feel the fact that we are drowning in fear, self-pity, doubt, anger, and sorrows. All we do by binge drinking is put our troubles off until tomorrow's retoxification. This is why we need supportive friends who will receive our wailing, miserable telephone calls. They better be good at listening, because drunken moaning is tedious. Don't ever call an ex and claim to be sober! Call mom or dad or someone like that, but have supportive relationships outside of those people too. Get supportive friends! What drives the drinking? What's with the emotional outbursts? Maybe, uhh...seek some fucking answers.

Falling: Up and down stairs, we fall both ways. While walking on the level ground our own damn goofy feet have betrayed us and left us flat on our face. What unnecessary pain we place on our face when drinking. We've had both our knees bleeding, bashed and bruised from last-night's unknown circumstances. Many fine jackets have been ruined. We fall off train platforms and tumble down the aisles on planes. We fall down in front of strangers and become one-time stars on YouTube. Strangers and the internet are really not so bad; it's when we fall down right in front of our children or girlfriends that it really hurts. We fall off barstools and think it's funny. We get thrown out of pubs and fall into gutters. We trip before the toilet and puke on the floor instead. We then sleep on the linoleum with our pants around our ankles. We stay lying in the rain because gravity is too hard to fight. Ah, drunkenness. Falling gets significantly more problematic with age.

Injuring: Of mysterious cuts and scrapes, we've all had our share. There've been burns, bloody gashes, broken bones, and clothes destroyed. But these are only minor consequences. Severe concussions can result from drinking far too much. Accidental death and vehicular manslaughter come to mind as well. These mistakes can change life forever and we bring these sorrows on ourselves by being drunk and careless. Self-inflicted injuries occur when conducting dangerous business without precaution, proper training, and attention. These preventative virtues fly right out the window when men get drunk. Naturally drunks are prone to inflicting injuries upon themselves. Drunks die and get crippled, but they also cause irreversible damage to others by their undisciplined behaviour. Some will lose their fingers and others their whole family. All alcohol related injuries are preventable, dumbass.

Violence: My fist has never visited another person's face, but I think I remember at least one time where my face was visited in such a fashion. Do you see a lot of sober fist fights? Sobriety is the only state in which conflict resolution can take place. Drinking and conflict are toxic buddies. Aggression is how men demand conformity within their male peer groups, but generally aggression enforces one-way agreements. It's mean. When we are the recipient of aggression or violence, a fight or flight response occurs, but there is also a paralysis response. Crisis response or bystander intervention is a wingding worth looking into. In a crisis tap into your breathing, and either lend a hand or get to safety.

Policing— we get arrested for drinking too much. We make these random friends and really attach to them. Isn't it fucked up how easy it is to get drunk with other drunks and try to drink everything before three A.M. Then what? Wander off to find some more! This hopeless quest can lead to more liquor being found, some cocaine, or a crazy argument with our new-found drinking buddies. If ya'll keep yelling and threatening each other, pretty soon the neighbors will call in a squad car. They'll arrest whomever they catch and throw 'em in the brightest, most cramped cell they've got: the drunk tank. In the middle of the floor there'll be a man breathing bubbles into a lake of his own piss. There'll also be young guys in jerseys sitting unimpressed, making stupid jokes. And there'll be completely uninteresting adult men just milling about. You'll get released pretty late in the day if you're arrested after midnight. Meditate, power through it. Try not to make it worse. Years later, you'll realize you learned something.

I bet you've done worse, or are just as bad. Address the regret, or intrusive thoughts will come up at inopportune moments. An example of intrusive thoughts would be like thinking about that puddle of piss while having a blowjob. Intrusive thoughts are major erection killers and cause invisible mood fluctuations.

Forgive yourself. Likely, the people you fucked over won't ever speak with you again. Whatever, that's sad, but there's no need to feel worse. Learn and grow, my man. Here are some tips for the terrible drunks:

Step 1: Stop drinking? Hell no, no way, not at this time. If you think you should stop, you should. Enlist in sobriety support. If you intend to keep drinking, acknowledge that drunken outbursts are a sign of needing (sober) emotional support—fact. What is going on there, buddy? Is drinking a means to cope with stress, anxiety, loss, or a lack knowing what else to do?

Step 2: Drink with people you know. Nothing says trouble like getting wasted with strangers. Alcohol tends to break down boundaries, fast. Generally, respecting boundaries is the only way to get to know folks better. New people are easier to offend than people who are familiar with our brand of idiocy.

Step 3: Know your limit. At some point, make the decision to stop drinking. If you are like me, you might find this difficult. Switch to water as soon as you feel drunk, bring less money, and cut yourself off earlier rather than later. This can extend the fun of an evening substantially and prevent puking, falling, and other painful embarrassments. Some temperance also prevents late-night limp-dick.

Step 4: After midnight. Get home soon after midnight to save yourself from transforming into a jackass like an evil Cinderella. When wasted, tired, and dehydrated, our dicks are either non-functional or underperforming anyways. Hanging around downtown after midnight is great way to find trouble, not sex.

The safety phrase "drink responsibly" is just a liability waiver—it basically says this is your own goddamn problem douche bag. In fact, advertisements, media, and our culture blatantly encourage men to drink excessively. Despite the sage precaution of "drink responsibly," every day millions of gallons of alcohol continue to drive our mediocrity and lethargy. We continue to be exhausted and stupefied, using temperance only as an afterthought. Smarten the fuck up. We can continue to hurt ourselves forever by our drinking, it's only when we hurt other people do we get attention. Unfortunately men are mostly silent about alcohol abuse; it is so pervasive and deeply entrenched in western masculine rituals. Resist the urge to become a drunken, stupid male. Formulate unique ideas about what fun looks like. This is far more appealing to woman, families, and law enforcement.

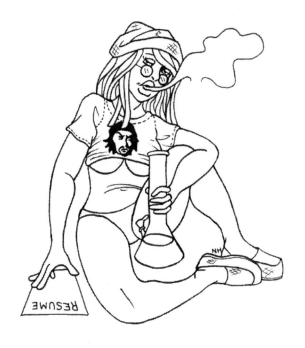

21.

Pfft, Stoners

How truly popular is marijuana? Is a one gram a day weed habit tough to kick? The withdrawal doesn't involve scratching off scabs so whatever, right? I'm pretty sure that when we get off the pot, the most likely withdrawal symptoms will be craving to get high again, boredom, anxiety, a lack of automatic dopamine, and lingering clarity.

Quite content to sit around all day eating snacks, pot smokers don't get out enough. We've got great ideas, but lack the initiative to actually do them. Pot smokers believe that lots of people smoke pot. Fortunately, this isn't true. Most people don't smoke weed, or if they do, they do so infrequently. However, when we only hang out with weed smokers, our world seems full of them. Confusion and removed contemplation is the natural state of pot smokers. When we smoke, we fall out of sync with the majority of our community and are left on the backbenches reflecting on life (rather than participating). It's awkward to communicate with people who aren't stoned. The general population makes us nervous. When we do finally get the courage to go outside, we're out of touch with the frequencies of ordinary folks. Not everyone thinks pot is as cool as stoners do.

Is pot a great drug for apathy? Is bong-smoking and non-voting related? Stoners will sit, smoke, and think long and hard about the virtues of conscientious objection, but do they make it to the polling station on voting day? Once dank goes legal, will all those highly vocal cannabis advocates quietly go away forever? Will they neglect to vote and forget the value of community participation? My fear is that stoners will be content on their balconies alone indefinitely, watching the world die with a glassy-eyed grin that suggests our doom was foretold—and they are alright with that.

When we live in a fatigued and cloudy state of mind, accomplishing things becomes a hassle. Advocates for marijuana will stop advocating after legalization because they'll need to have a long nap—that's when corrupted corporations will step in. If pot advocates could fix the grungy aesthetics of cannabis culture, they would get more respect. The problem is that self-medicating and self-diagnosis will lead to unmanaged side effects. As a chronic pot smoker, respect is hard to come by. The stoner is a victim of stigma. Certain professional positions will not be available. Cannabis use will strain relationships. Here are a few things to prevent becoming a burn-out:

Don't wear stupid hats—Don't be so damn unhygienic looking—Don't wear global colours and claim to understand their significance—Don't praise political figures whose history you can't articulate—Don't speak to the media and demonstrate worse speaking skills than a teenage prom queen—Don't wear tinted glasses—Don't eat Cheetos while discussing the health benefits of weed—Don't buy corn-syrup-based candy and claim to believe in locally sourced, organic, GMO free, and fair trade stuff—Don't accumulate pizza boxes, take-out containers, fast food wrappers, and energy drinks in your foyer—Don't pretend you can stop whenever you want—Don't ignore the compounding social problems that marijuana creates—Don't think of weed as a cure for pain, anxiety, or depression, it is a temporary respite at best—Don't smoke around children—Don't say marijuana helps you cope with real life problems.

I am eager for marijuana to be medically legalized. Then we can address the underlying problems that drive us to smoke it. Like, why are we self-medicating? Are there better solutions? How are the side-effects impacting our lives? Men are notorious for never seeing a doctor. With medical oversight cannabis legalization presents an opportunity to open avenues to address men's health like never before. Cannabis should not become like the alcohol industry. Under the cloud of weed smoke, men are coping with their problems alone, in a fashion that doesn't jeopardize their masculine identity. Understand this: we *are* self-medicating. Why? How? When? What for?

Men are possibly medicating for depression, rage, nerve damage, knee pain, social-isolation, head injury, neck injury, loneliness, boredom, alcohol abuse, trauma, divorce, stress, fear, suicide, and probably a lot of other stuff too. The point being, stoners have real life problems on top of their coping methods being criminalized. Let's deal with cannabis use in an open and direct fashion by being proactive about men's health prevention. There are tons of feelings that we're numbing with weed. Ask supporters to help you move on from this prevalent depressant. Binge drinking and bong hits are a terrible primary means to cope. It's just so unoriginal.

Lasting good feelings don't come from reefer. If this is how you cope, acknowledge the medicinal property seriously and the side-effects. Weed won't make us excited, hopeful, and full of life, but it will gloss over our mental and physical health symptoms quite effectively. That's the perk of a daily dose of dope: medicating our dissatisfaction. Here some steps to consider:

> Step 1: Few smoke. The vast majority of people do not smoke pot regularly. By association, you exist in an isolated social realm of like-minded individuals. All of whom (yourself included) are

having difficulties with real life problems. Instead of budgeting and future planning, you can expect a candy habit, under-employment, and impulse buys. The snacks, the weed, and the video gaming are all representative of you being stuck in a rut that could go on forever.

Step 2: Chubby. Pot smokers aren't known for their athleticism. Some significant downsides to cannabis deserve attention. These include the constant consumption of sweet and salty snacks, staying up late playing video games, mid-day lethargy, staying inside all day, aversion to exercise, skipping breakfast, and not packing a lunch. These are just a few behaviours pot smokers display.

Step 3: Men. It is mostly men who smoke pot and I'd wager that most women are introduced to cannabis by men. If you are going to keep up this habit for the rest of your life, you better recognize that you might be a lonely, lazy dude who is hiding his emotional bullshit with drugs.

Step 4: Addiction. We get addicted to cannabis. Let's not lie to ourselves for a hundred years like we did with tobacco. Blanket proof is simple: is it more pleasant to be stoned than not? An entrenched cannabis habit will crave the return to that stoned state repeatedly. The happy-relaxed feeling that cannabis can provide masks the truth of the dependency and our fragile emotional state.

Cannabis is on the way to becoming marginally acceptable. Its emergence requires temperance, community support, and research initiatives in order to make legalization a positive healthcare step in our communities. As a medicine, cannabis today presents one of the most accessible points of entry to provide healthcare services to young men and develop their long term prevention plans.

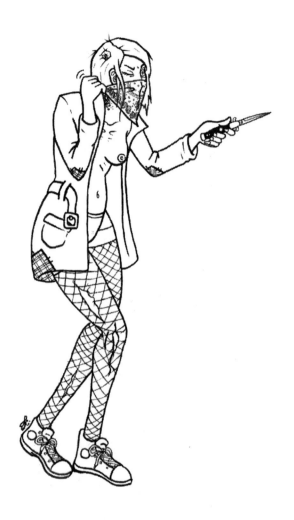

22.
Hard-Ass Fucking Drugs and Robbery

There are hard-ass fucking drugs out there that will change our lives forever, never for the better. What begins as good times and rattling vibrations can end up as unabashedly addictive behaviour, dangerous lifestyles, and shameless emotional denial.

I've put down a synopsis of some hard drugs that we might have ingested over the years:

Psychedelics: Avoid operating motor vehicles and heavy equipment when using these kinds of drugs (and all drugs). You need someone to take care of you on this kind of trip. They are your spirit guide, so listen to them. Bad trips require hyperventilation treatment and possibly hospitalization. A teddy bear is comforting and can do a lot for bringing down a bad trip. Drug bender freak-outs can happen to anyone and may lead to screaming, raving, death, and insanity. When the police eventually pick you up, you might get a trip to the local psychiatric ward. It depends on three factors. How naked were you? Have you suddenly developed a newfound belief in aliens? How long does the psychosis last for?

By taking these drugs, we steer ourselves into mental/emotional fatigue and become isolated from our community. Though we might believe we are a sage and pilgrim soul, our magic powers are undeniably lacking. The shiny lights of the world will over-stimulate our brains and make any clear direction impossible. One day, all those shiny lights, including ours, will burn out. We will have forgotten a great deal and been left to rediscover ourselves without trippin' balls.

Narcotics: Can we stop the drug war if we stop buying? Maybe, but I think it requires narcotics users to actually read a book and learn new stuff. It is hard to claim to be a real man when we have a chemical addiction stronger than our sex drive. This chemical dicklessness makes the male user very angry. To compensate, he is aggressive and agitated. These are scary kinds of fuckos. His cock and balls have been shrivelled up for hours, and I'm sober, charming and capable of fucking tonight. He is jealous of svelte men, because he can't get his dick up or speak coherently. Using his outside voice while inside is how the narcotics compensate his manliness in this setting. This shit will fuck up our children, hurt our families, and drive the man into aggressive extremes due to repeat rejection. These folks need help and don't have any fucking clue how to get it.

Steroids: Do not believe beauty magazines; they make us feel ugly. Also, they have created those charmingly aggressive men who take steroids in order to fit rigorous physical ideals of manliness. These men make the most difficult coworkers. The perks of their musculature is corroded by their volatility and ghastly social skills. They are ugly on the inside. Bystanders can see the connection between their physique and shitty temperament as by-products of their vanity drug. Like all drug-users, they will find themselves surrounded by others similar to them. Through osmosis, their peer group excuses the physical pain in their testicles as an acceptable side-effect. Jacked-up testosterone combined with rampant dick pain results in a negative mental environment for a dude, hey? Couple that with some drunken stupidity, a ferocious sex-drive *sans* erection, and we have a scary group of drug addicts. These blue-balled backscratchers were never told they were smart, so they choose to look strong. Though athletes can be intelligent, they cannot be if they are taking steroids and risking their health. All they do is set their bodies up for disaster. What will they do then? Men wouldn't take steroids without extreme vanity; at what cost and to what extent will we strive for an ideal physical body? Where would we be without it? Happy?

New Age Smack: Don't dabble in this shit, kids. People on chemical drugs are impossible to handle—it's like killing ourselves slowly. When we do get clean, we will not be the same person we were. Not by a long shot. Chances are that if we are using these drugs we never bought this book and our reading comprehension is shit. With severe chemical addictions, imagine howling. Stealing from your family. Suffering all kinds of abuse. Being delirious, confused, angry, and desperate. On the streets every night. Afraid of our addicted, thieving friends: an underground network of people we distrust. Cold and tense. Cigarettes to numb the withdrawal. Constipation and self-loathing. Hopelessness, suicide, desperation, and insomnia. Drug addiction is like a kind of vampirism. Our craving to feed, stay up at night, and risk all kinds of social villainy grows with each feeding, but instead of having fangs, our teeth are rotting, our face is sagging, and we've become distanced from anyone who cares.

Be wary of people on hard-ass fucking drugs. They may be nice people but desperation is a cruel master. At some point, they will need money for another hit. Where does the money come from? I wouldn't want to be around to find out. How we answer the following question determines where we're at:

Would you prefer:
A) crack, heroin, or meth B) a soup & sandwich C) both, bitch!

To qualify as a borderline criminal drug-user, the correct answer is C. A indicates that we're still new to the lifestyle and not quite opportunistic enough yet. Hard-ass fucking drug users aren't criminals or robbers or accidental murderers necessarily, but poverty, helplessness, and addiction are dire motivators.

Solutions for poverty must become a national priority. Our lack of common economic support spurs incredible suffering. Substance abuse is indicative of generations of trauma, community malaise, and unaddressed mental health problems. Poverty is a traumatic mental health problem. Society ignores this at its own peril. If we have an addiction and haven't got a healthy community support system, we have a mental health problem. Isolation will compound our barriers to recovery. Understand that all users are doing the best they can to cope. Don't give up trying; it will take everything we've got, plus support to recover. People do recover.

Now, a few tips regarding the subject of hard drugs.

Step 1: Don't. This one is pretty straightforward. We've heard it a lot. And really, abstinence-based recovery is ideal. By getting clean and not using drugs, we might recover our friends and family. Love is prevented by our love of getting high. Lots of good things come to those who don't use hard drugs.

Step 2: Help. When we see a friend on a path of self-destruction, help them. Offer help often. Drill them and keep coming back to them. Nag them. Give them tons of support. Keep calling. Say affirming words like "keep trying," "what can I do," and "I believe in you." Tell them to put your number in their phone and call if they are in a crisis. Friendships will be strained by the use of hard drugs, and you may not be able to help someone. Be prepared to set boundaries when friends go toxic, but always keep hope alive for them, even if you can no longer support them.

Step 3: Estrangement. The worst thing about these kinds of drugs is how supporters will be driven away. Long-term support is hard to find anyways, and drugs make it much more difficult because our social circles are so constrained. When a drug habit has estranged us from our good friends and our family, we need to dump our addicted buddies and check into a recovery centre. Connection is a key to recovery.

Step 4: Recovery. Check in for help. Go see a doctor. Getting re-incarcerated is not the answer to the long-term reclamation of our lives. Use every resource available in your town to get clean. Imagine a future vision of yourself and commit it to writing. This is the new you. Work towards getting there. Set reasonable, attainable goals, and scale them up over time. This is the process of becoming a new man. It's fun and scary. Apply patience and compassion for yourself.

Circumstances of your life will lead you into frightening situations. One of those situations could be serious drug addiction. Without curbing your serious addictions, positive relationships will be virtually impossible.

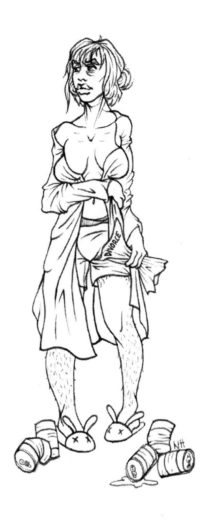

23.

So You Fucked It All Up...

It is the worst, most utterly terrible moment when we realize that we are directly responsible for another person's misery. Yes, sometime our actions can cause immense distress in someone close to us. Their response could come in the form of screaming, tears, icy silence, or police involvement. What did we do to elicit such domestic strife? Maybe we fell down the stairs, crashed the car, lost our job, or flipped into a rage. Berserk behaviour responses, though incredibly stimulating, never leads to sex, happiness, or solutions. When we calm down, it always comes back through either reprimand or abandonment. If we get punished for stupid behaviour, or dumped it's because we will probably do it all over again.

Fucking up repeatedly shows how badly we treat ourselves. It is never someone else's fault when we fuck up. Right up to the moment of morning-after consciousness, everything is just dandy. When we discover ourselves situated comfortably on the bathroom floor with a blanket and pillow, something bad probably happened. Unconsciousness seems like heaven compared to a dry mouth and a vague sense of dread. That may be the last night of you having a wife. In the kitchen, she has neatly arranged the beer bottles just enough to make her hand-written divorce note easy to find.

Well done; it's over. We might have to miss work for a day after a major fuck up. This moment of crisis can go okay or very bad. How we handle ourselves in this moment will more-or-less determine the trajectory of our recovery. Resist the post-divorce abyss, and try to push towards stability and emotional acceptance. A positive transformation is beginning: from a totally fucked up douche bag to decent human male (like a fucking butterfly). Grieve, lonely man. Fumble about home like a zombie. Try in vain and make it better. Become more deeply miserable and realize that this isn't going to get better overnight.

Unfortunately it's on us, the drug soaked douche bags, to fix our shit. Oh god, I wish it wasn't the case. I wish there was a quick fix, but frankly, the odds are against men even identifying their basic sadness and confusion. Why do men fuck shit up so much? Who is doing this to us? Men are essentially good, but when life requires emotional discomfort, men tend to behave unusually aggressively. It is as if emotions are so confusing to men that we feel a need to attack them. It appears that men are afraid of feelings and would prefer to continue fucking up than to help themselves.

Enter emotional numbing. When we fuck it all up, we'll try binge drinking with buddies at least once. They'll inject us with alcohol because they don't know how to deal with our feelings any better than we do. Between drinks, they'll subject us to a number of clichés, which won't help: "You're better than her," "You'll find someone," "Let's go find you another," "What a bitch." Such phrases are useful for buddies because they acknowledge but simultaneously avoid understanding the central feelings. Buddies wait for the beer to gloss over us until we are happy with our alcohol level, at which point they resort to their pattern friendship strategies such as sport fucking or stupid head games. Good luck love-fucking while drinking to misery.

When you fuck it all up, and you will, avoid compounding the problem. This includes combining divorce with disastrous behaviours like binge-drinking, fighting, and driving across town for a row with your ex. Men should fuck up sometimes. It is a rite of passage for a man to be at the epicenter of a power-ful event at least once, just don't get anyone hurt. Understand that the act of trying necessitates some failing. Get accustomed to small errors, avoid big ones by learning. Learn from those who have fucked up before us: try, fail, recover, and try again. One step forward and one step back is a handy dance step too. But when shit-tastic setbacks happen, we triple the size of the shit-sling if we react like an emotionally immature jackass.

Hopefully we don't just keep repeating the same patterns forever, thinking that some mystery women will eventually love us unconditionally. I doubt that is going to work. Mom is figuratively dead. Recover from childhood. Don't forsake it—keep curiosity, wonder, and playfulness. Have the feelings, and let 'em fly—articulated. No tantrums.

Never take a tissue when you cry. Blow your nose on your right sleeve and wipe your eyes with the left. I just want you to give a shit about yourself and see your shortcomings as your own damn responsibility. Here are some fucking tips to stop fucking up so much.

Step 1: Avoid prison. Fucking things up extends to the entire range of a man's existence. If you wind up imprisoned from poor emotional control, a time out is certainly called for. That being said, ordinary men (of the non-prison variety) benefit from alone time and self-reflection. This opportunity is in abundance whilst incarcerated.

Step 2: Apologize sincerely. If you have realized how greatly you've fucked everything up, chances are you are beating yourself up quite badly. Take your time making your apology because, in the early moments of realization, you don't yet fully know what you are apologizing for. Drink in the full scope of the damage you did, sleep on it, and man-up for a long drawn-out conversation. Apologizing many times will deteriorate your confidence and the relationship equity. One good apology is better than ten meek ones.

Step 3: Forgive yourself quietly. If you find that you are berating yourself days after an incident, ask why. It's not necessary to be gloomy if you've learned something. Just don't brag that you've recovered when really you've just fallen back into the same shit. That's denial. Try to get back on your A-game. If you stay down on yourself, negative choices will avail themselves more frequently. Forgive yourself and begin daily routines that will reduce the odds of fucking up again.

Step 4: Lose with grace. When everything is lost, do it with grace. Come up with a plan for when the shit hits the fan. Here is what to do when everything is going fucking terrible:

A: Remain calm, do not lash out.
B: Retreat from triggers.
C: Contact supporters.
D: Make a man plan.

Many men of better quality than you have fucked everything up. Men become infamous for it. However, when properly handled, women find a man of action (who tries, fails, and recovers) infinitely more attractive than a man who never tries or stays miserable. If you feel you've got nothing going for you right now, I suggest you take up volunteering in your community. You will discover that healthy masculinity is needed in our neighborhoods and schools.

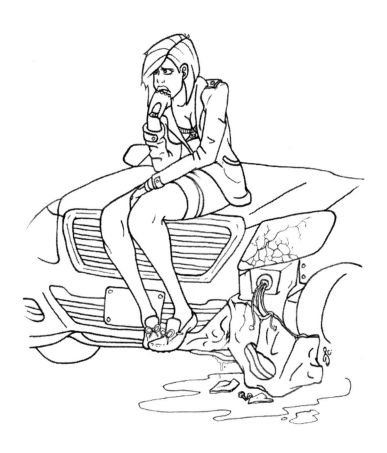

24.
Hating Yourself Should Be Temporary and Contextual

I like me. Say it with me: I like me. I like me. Despite the obvious cheesiness, being kind to ourselves will help. Too bad we don't just start conversations with sincere compliments, hey? Well, we don't because it wouldn't be very genuine. We tend to be competitive in our assessment of other men. The result of this kind of toxic masculinity includes shame for our (plentiful) shortcomings, defensiveness, arrogance, and aggression. The truth is, however, that a healthy ego requires lots of energy and self-reflection to sustain, and it is not without self-doubt.

Coming off as arrogant is never ideal. Arrogance is confidence under attack. It highlights our sense of our entitlement and our emotional masking. Why do we need arrogance? What have we done lately to jeopardize people's confidence in us? Something, I'm sure. Our body language informs nearby folks about our bravado and the emotional walls we've set up. Male body language is particularity noticeable and, because of men's minimal emotional output, men are easy to predict. Physical restriction suggests mental tension. Too often men are unknowingly emotionally triggered; that ignorance makes him susceptible to intrusive thoughts and reactionary hostility. This permeates in his appearance, judgement and condescension show on his face. With that much mental energy being channeled into hostile appearances, how can men possibly stay focused, positive, and hopeful? Our anger and distrust is super fucking toxic and we inflict it upon ourselves. To help this go away we have to honour the context of our anger and trust that it can be a temporary emotional state. Self-esteem is created by our track record, resilience, and recovery—not set-backs, not self-pity, and never violence.

Recovery from failure sucks, but if we let ourselves be defeated by it (and not learn from it), then we'll wind up meek and wimpy. There are unspoken assessments exchanged instantly between men while passing in the street. If we have repeatedly failed to recover from failures, other men will detect our ineptitude through our body language. What I'm saying is that we subconsciously assess men on their level of threat in a way that we don't generally do with women. The man who hates himself is a more likely victim or perpetrator of domestic violence. If a man has little value for his own life he will put less value in the lives of others. This is instantly detected in our subliminal analysis of other men. Hypothetically, any characteristic can be considered a threat. Our level of confidence in dealing with social threats is related to how much genuine confidence we have. Perceived threats need not be rational and can include sexuality, skin colour, tattoos, stature, bicep diameter, clothes, or quirkiness. Nowadays men can take preventative measures through lifestyle management and daily health maintenance to positively assert their masculinity and not risk as much marginalization as they did in the past. Behaviours of non-recovery (giving up or denial) and bravado (masking) are indicative of men without practice in resolving these social conflicts.

We're conditioned to walk it off and ignore our problems—it's shit. Society has manufactured men as emotionally restricted. Whatever, we're human cattle. Civilizations have savagely attempted to exterminate one another, even now. We are born pre-subjugated by our own ethnic histories and preconditioned with ideas of racism, prejudice, misogyny, and toxic masculinity. This shit it's also reinforced by how we chose to live our lives and what we teach our children. It does not always have to be this way. Breaking this cycle is the context of the era in which we now live. The information age has brought about massive global change. Accompanying that change involves men overcoming centuries of institutional conditioning that have solidified our masculine stupidity-norms.

There are two worst-case scenarios for rage-styled emotions: murder and suicide. This is why it is important to see that hating ourselves (and others) is always temporary and contextual. Violent folks have evolved from a long evolutionary history of unique challenges and a pattern of violent reactions. Let's pretend we are them for a moment. In this moment, we believe our immediate future is deadly and intense—we are going to kill someone right now. Inherently we feel hopelessness and rage but, due to stupid masculinity protocols, we repress it. We can only repress it for so long until we sincerely don't value our own lives; that's when fatal thoughts take hold. Then something else shitty happens (say, bankruptcy or divorce) and now we have even more problems. With no perceivable release from this anguish, a reasonable man can be pushed over the edge. What he fails to see is that this emotional state is temporary and contextual—life is long. The survivors of man's destructive rage are left wondering what the fuck they could have done to prevent it: educate men in emotional intelligence, healthcare prevention, and talk about suicide.

We can understand ourselves better by compartmentalizing our personal history in order to highlight when our self-esteem got punched in the mouth. When did our self-esteem even begin? Can we remember the first time we felt embarrassed? How do we react to conflicts? Do we shrink and fear other people? Do we become hostile when we perceive a challenge? How do we think the world see us?

My first experience of "being seen," or terrible embarrassment, was nothing short of triumphant. Except for the boy named Shannon, he didn't get off so lucky.

I was in Grade 2. I had an environmentalist for a teacher so she had us do a nature play for the student talent showcase. Seems appropriate, right? All the kids were given butterfly-shaped sheets of paper. The students painted only one side of the paper wings and then we folded the wings in half to imprint a symmetrical pattern on them. I'm sure it was delightful. That Friday was the performance. My class all wore black for the skipping and frolicking (to Enya) in the gymnasium with our painted paper wings. This presentation of interpretative dance required two students to read a one-page handout into the microphone before the whole school (with parents in attendance). A boy named Shannon and I were selected. When we got on stage, poor little Shannon peed himself and ran off crying. Meanwhile I, alone on stage, decided to read the whole damn handout. That is the moment I became addicted to applause.

But all egos and environments are not created equally. Self-esteem certainly fluctuates.

> Step 1: Poor Shannon. Our ability to speak before a crowd is not improving with technology. Public speaking will feel uncomfortably exhilarating and we'll be left feeling like we could have done better. Keep practicing. Ride that excitement. It is difficult to be seen standing out but it is necessary for men to speak out when they witness injustices—this is how we will save ourselves. Will the modern man have the confidence to advocate for himself, his spouse, or his community with so little practice? Will men fail their duty as able-bodied citizens to make positive change? When men witness conflict do they freeze, shrink, or hide? When immediate action is vital, will men be clear minded and act accordingly for what is right and just? Will he forgive himself if he fails to act? If there's doubt or fear, remember: it is temporary and contextual. Shannon had nothing to fear except the emotion of fear. Masculinity is blessed by its ability to make an impact, so make it good. In those life-defining split-second moments, breathe deeply and respond with your heart. Silence and our failure to engage

contributes massively to our own health decline. It is the fuel of an apathetic culture rife with narcissism, wholesale cowardice, and self-gratification at the expense of others. Speaking is not a grand gesture. We all have an inner voice and can use it to do what is right, regardless if we've fucked up in the past.

Step 2: Situational confidence. Don't just jump up on stage and embarrass yourself, leave that to professionals. Take a speech class if you want to improve your diction, comprehension, and spoken flexibility—speaking is an extremely useful skill that can be improved. Nevertheless, you already have confidences. What are they? Are they appealing or useful? Are they inclusive of your community? Will your potential father-in-law value your skill set?

Step 3: Never deny ignorance. Gas is too expensive to drive around the goddamn block for another twenty minutes. Ask for directions! Set your flaws free, gentlemen. Feel free to learn new skills while you are doing it. That's what being a man is about: doing stuff, then doing more stuff, and then having a nap. Likely you cannot safely operate power tools and serenade a lover. You're probably uncomfortable dancing so you never try, and you've watched a lot of porn but don't quite get how to fuck yet. These are all workable problems! Recognize those blind spots.

Step 4: Recover from it. You are gonna be you no matter what. You are you. I am me. Mom is Mom and Cynthia is gonna be Cynthia. You have got to be you because everyone else is taken. Effort is the only actual solution available if you want to improve, sucker. Put effort in and get over the traumas, get over the rejections, and get over your fear of learning. Meditation is great, get a mentor, and finish your projects. Setting milestones (even negative ones) is a great way to track change.

Exercise your inner strength. It's in there. Find it monthly. Every fucking month try rediscovering some motivation. Constantly be failing at something so that you know what it feels like to build back up again. Care about the fucking changes that you're fucking trying to make, damnit. It's not always going to work out perfectly.

Hey, at least we're trying.

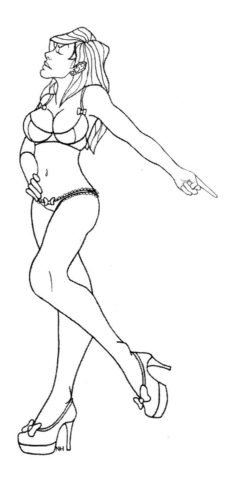

25.
Blaming Others and
Avoiding Responsibility

The only thing better than getting away with a guilty pleasure, is witnessing someone get busted. It's like getting blackmailed by a pimp after a blowjob. "Mhm, damn that was so good. Shh, oh, wait. What? Oh shit, did you just photograph me? Who the fuck is that guy? What? Fuck you, what do you mean you know my wife? How do you know my name? I'm not giving you any fucking money... Oh...okay...just calm down...put the fucking knife down. Fine, here's the money. Fucker. Shit! Okay. I'm leaving. I'm leaving! Ow! God damnit! You fucker, you hit me right in the mouth. Asshole."

Good luck explaining that.

"Where did you get that bruise? What were you doing last night? You don't look very good. Not again! What the fuck happened to your face? Why the fuck are you doing this to yourself? What? It's my fault? You say it's my fault? You are out of your fucking mind. Get out, you fucking asshole! Fuck you! Get out!"

I don't know why men make such risky choices and try to wiggle out of the consequences. I don't know why we get so defensive or why we rage like maniacs. All I know is that, whatever the reasons, it's certainly some unresolved personal problem spilling out into the community. Yes, capitalism sucks and that shit is stressful. Yes, mass media has portrayed men as stupid, stone-faced sex villains. And yes, a man's life is subjugated to the winds of politics and warfare. There is a lot to rage against! Misery abounds. Shall we repress our anger and suffer internally, or let it fly?

Let it fly! Just don't hurt anyone. Find outlets. The repression of negative emotions has the effect of repressing all emotions. That numbness creates a sense of purposelessness.

Use patient, systematic, and logical releases for aggressiveness. Every man is poisoned with some aggressive tendencies. We hide it at the expense of others and our own sanity. Those who manage their aggression can identify, embrace, and pacify their anger before it comes out as aggressive volatility. Work through aggressive urges with someone trustworthy and hash out how to identify aggressive emotions before they erupt. This may prevent self-destructive behaviours, curtail our fuckups, and reduce our need to use scapegoats and blame.

Shirking responsibility, especially when we have hurt people, lowers our value in the community, workplaces, and relationships. The guilt surrounding taking responsibility isn't permanent. It may be uncomfortable, but is an emotional path to better integrity. Never over-apologize or become meek; however, if we seek soft-skinned company in our senior years, practice conflict resolution every day. In relationships we make promises (ie: respect, decency, and kindness) and breaking them is easy when we have a habit of avoid consequences. Restoration and forgiveness vary depending on the severity of the fuckup, but avoidance makes recovery impossible.

When we stubbornly hold onto self-righteousness, it becomes difficult to get along with others. This is easier said than done because we are deeply committed to our patterns and beliefs, even if they offer us little benefit. Imagine if religious zealots suddenly gave up and said, "Oops, we've been wrong forever. Circumcision is kinda weird, and God is sorry for cutting off part of your penis." That will probably never happen. We can't ask haters to stop hating without asking believers to stop believing. Don't have beliefs, have feelings. Preachers are like gang affiliates in how entrenched their philosophies lay. For a man to change, say from an angry mobster to a healthy supportive father, he must invalidate a part of how he has lived his entire life. It means he wasn't living the way he wanted and he was wrong for decades. Fact. Stepping away from our old self is a matter of behavioural awareness. All we've gotta do is trim up and stop blaming PE teachers and bullies for our own rickety bones.

It takes effort to change old patterns. We have to completely accept that we follow an uncertain trajectory, we don't have all the answers, and that our goal is to stop loss. Bad shit happened. It hurt for a long time. It's confusing for a long time too. But when we fuck up, we've got to rally supporters and get some personal insight. Self-advocacy, my man! It requires that we talk about ourselves and learn our unmet needs. Conflict resolution helps us take responsibility for our actions and recover with some grace. It's never too late to start new patterns.

We are men under renovation. We've got a foundation that'll last for possibly three generations to come. We are hiring a crew of workers inside our minds to retrofit our original construction and accommodate future occupants. We will receive seismic upgrades, and solar panels for improved stability and energy efficiency. We will become capable of emotional risks and recharge in the sunshine.

Here are some steps to less blame.

Step 1: Weather storms. Categorize, acknowledge, and re-story the moments you have suffered greatest. You don't have to go chasing conflicts. Retroactively set milestones where you can identify personal change. From a place of accepting your past shit-storm, make future engagements that set you up to succeed despite odds. Thriving regardless of adversity is called resiliency.

Step 2: Avoid blame. Short of being earnestly fucked over by someone or identifying crooks, generally it's best to bear the burden of our past with a conscious effort to overcome life's challenges. When troubles get too heavy, however, take a rest and ask for help. Despite what philosophers might say, you have free will and can make choices. External forces are not totally responsible for our happiness, our own choices are.

Step 3: Responsibility. Sometimes we must even take responsibility for events beyond our control. When external forces put pressure on us, we have a duty to respond in a non-violent fashion. Historically men are the great movers of mountains; the penetrators of the sea and sky. Men have wielded more fire than any creature to have ever existed on Earth. Marvel at the aftermath of man. We are responsible for the generational changes we have made, for better or worse, consciously or not. This reckless abandon is only trumped in depravity by apathetic hopelessness. We cannot just diddle ourselves and play pretend war games without seeing the isolation and limited intellectual perspective that our entertainment offers. Minds occupied with false deaths will become desensitized to the impact of violence until it literally hits us in the face. This artificial aggression or violence at a distance, makes minor acts of cruelty in real life seem insignificant. This fallacy builds over time as we repeatedly dismiss malevolent behaviours as normal. Harbouring ill will is the irresponsible choice to not resolve, not feel better, and not recover from conflict. It moves men further away from contentiousness, connections with their local communities, and sex.

Step 4: Oops, pregnancy. Baby-daddy syndrome is a violent fucking plague. First, what the fuck are men doing barebacking women they don't wanna impregnate? Give me a fucking break. That is not how a decent man approaches his generational continuity. Wear a goddamned fucking condom. Fifteen minutes (or less) of a silky, wet, naked pussy are not worth a massive life-altering event like babies or sexually transmitted infections. Stop fucking up the gene pool, morons. Prior to barebacking, date a woman for a couple of cycles, go get simultaneously tested, add monogamy, add birth control, and go at it for as long as it lasts. Great sex takes trust and repeat performances. We can hurt other people (for generations) when we fuck like idiots, so sort it out, dipshit.

Well, now you know. It's you. It is your fault that you keep making the same mistakes. You can complain and deflect forever but it's a lot more effective if you make a plan. Professional help can be super fucking useful. In isolation, recovery is impossible. By smartening the fuck up and owning our actions, we become way cooler.

If men can develop some emotional intelligence, internal and external conflict need not necessitate aggression.

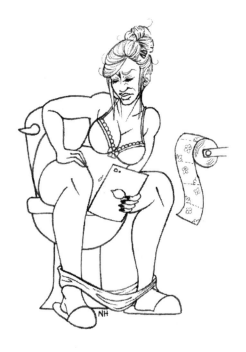

26.

Poop's Great, Especially When Your Asshole Doesn't Bleed

Oh man, you know it's true: pushing a nice big semi-soft shit out your backend feels fantastic.

When was the last time we bragged about our shits? It was either the last time our moms fed us vegetables or when a shit was so satisfying it was worthy of gossip. Man-themed parties (like the Super Bowl) aren't packed with foods conducive to great shits, but they are packed with men who appreciate a good shit. That appreciation suggests that a good poop might be a novelty, not a regular perk. Here are some reasons why Sports fans waddle while they walk: treacherous gas, constipation, batwings, an insufficiently wiped ass, or microscopic anal lacerations. This does not exclude the co-occurrence of moist, chafing, hairy thighs—or injury.

Men swagger because they've recently pooped or need to poop. They may even have tiny scabs around their anuses that have not healed. Guys, wiping harder does not make the bleeding stop. You can try applying lotions to your asshole and you can dab it with some cool water. Try seeing a doctor for that swagger. At the end of your colonoscopy, the proctologist will say, "Eat less processed food, candy, and beer," among other, more doctorly, insights.

Colonoscopy: getting your butt penetrated by a doctor and his big gay camera. Uncomfortable? Yes. Arousing? Unlikely. Regardless, this is called vital health care prevention. We can start early by not shitting out Cheetos and poorly chewed steaks. A poop should be a pleasant experience for a man. Poop is nature's barometer to assess the efficiency of our intestines without invading our homo-aggressive assholes with a camera on a bendy cord.

When it isn't a good poop, take notes. Keep a poop chart, I dare you. Assess the enjoyment of the experience, and cross-reference it to what you've been jamming down your pie hole for the last day. Taking note of your shit could help you understand your health better. All from the convenience of your toilet bowl!

For the experienced pooper, I would like to suggest some advanced tips. Squat, if your flexibility permits it. Use your breath. Be patient. Use slow and consistent pressure. Don't rush by pushing too hard. Support bars are available for those physically exhausting shits. Also, the toilet paper can really make or break the experience. The bidet is a lost treasure. When pooping among company don't pretend to sneak off to the bathroom like nobody noticed—you were gone for too long for it to be only a piss. When in restaurants, be sure to laugh heartily when the guy in the next stall farts loudly and moans heavily, the laugh will help your evacuation. Farts are funny, but also may indicate disharmony in the rectum.

If you've got regular sharts (self-soiling farts), daily gut pain, seepage, or shit blood (not to be mistaken with having eaten beets), override your faith in WebMD and consult a real physician.

For not having uncomfortable poops:

Step 1: New things. International culinary experiences may cause disruptions in our bowels for the better. I suggest that we try new things to suss out an ideal shit schedule. A regiment of bland, sweet, and salty flavors has led us to an intolerance of real food. But can a man die by lack of spice? Maybe not, but hosting friends for dinner certainly fights off isolation. I know full-grown men who only eat meat, bread, potatoes, and sauce. They are single, unfriendly, chubby, and have poor skin. If we don't wish to look like a glistening ham, bow to the beauty of new things. Like vegetables and spices!

Step 2: Log your logs. Try this. Consistent poops are preferable. You ought to know what clogs you up or thins you out. If you want to see the effect your diet has on your body, look no further than the porcelain Petri dish in the bathroom. You will spend a significant portion of your life pressing crap out your ass, so you might as well track and cross-reference it with your food intake. Becoming aware of it will help. Charting your shitting experience will make a funny party joke and shed light on poop health.

Step 3: Dissection isn't necessary. Observation is okay, but don't handle your own feces. If this is a psychological thingy, you should probably seek help. If corn is clearly visible, maybe corn isn't working. Was it an enjoyable poop? Wonder, just wonder, what you consumed lately. Those BBQ chicken wings and beers are far less pleasant coming out than going in.

Step 4: Not for sharing. If you are competitor in your peer group for largest coiler, or if a buddy has literally shit in the tub and you want to blackmail him, photograph the shit. However, photographing shits and sharing it online is as gross as grannies with butt plugs. There are no cultures that think it's awesome to throw shit around (except monkeys). The only appropriate way to share crap is some eco-fertilizer movement.

Okay, this shit is over. The sooner we start tracking our diet and our poops, the better we'll adjust to shitting at the age when it becomes infinitely more difficult. Add tooth loss and our good shitting days are gone. The idiocy of fast food and soda pop wreaks havoc on our delicate sphincters.

Seek good poop solutions.

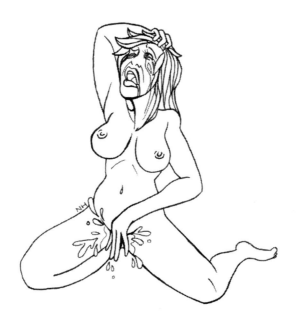

27.

Sex is Self-Esteem. Fortunately You Can Go Fuck Yourself

Good or bad, fact or fiction, it is generally said that men want a lot of sex. Fortunately, they can always go fuck themselves. It is simply not possible to have as much sex as we might imagine (see: population crisis).

Fucking yourself is an imitation of romance directed at the self. Make it special. Light a fucking candle, lie in bed, and summon mental images about your sex fantasies. Take your time; your sex moves are outdated and your imagination is rusty. Shit, your body isn't even accustomed to actual in-bed sex. Use only two fingers while you whack off. Vaginas are not as tight as your masturbatory death grip. Use lube, maybe even a fancy jelly stroker—it will simulate the proper pressure of a vagina. While you romantically stroke you own dick, imagine your partner is in the room or someone you have a crush on. What a concept! Thinking about a real woman you'd like to date, and who you've actually met. This may begin creating an urge to speak with said individual and perhaps ask them on a date. However, don't ever discuss the fact you whack off and think about them; that is private.

Lust respectfully. Fill yourself with admiration for your crush's intellectual qualities, the subtleties of their beauty, and the way they make you feel. Too often men fuck women and then go brag to their buddies to elevate their homosocial status. This man has pre-numbed himself to the fact that she will probably leave him. The overtly lusty male has a mediocre emotional capacity, and is in no shape for quality women. The satisfaction he seeks is male-male approval and not the satisfaction of an excellent shared experience within the context of a healthy sexual relationship. That guy should just go fuck himself.

When we want past lovers to come back, is it because we haven't found new ones yet? This is called bargaining. It's called bargaining when we want an expired relationship to return. This is being lazy, unoriginal, and not progressing. That's probably why she left. Go find greener pastures and try to learn from rejection. Mediocre rebound sex is not an anti-depressant. Don't use sex to impress douche bag friends. Having gossip-worthy sex will make a man more confident with sex, but bragging about it is a douche maneuver that seeks validation from the wrong people. To develop a strong sense of self-esteem, be available for special relationships so that when you fuck it all up, you'll know how to earn it again.

It's alright to feel depressed about getting dumped: sex is gone, your self-esteem is rocked, and you're forced back to fucking yourself. Be as miserable as possible as quickly as possible. Eat comfort food, see friends and family, sleep in, and call in sick. Do not pretend that everything is okay, or it'll be fine. Self-esteem should take a figurative beating occasionally. By shortcutting our feelings we demean our experience. If we say that we are fine when we are actually miserable, misery becomes our new normal. All of a sudden, happiness is much more difficult to achieve. Be miserable and angry, but don't lie and say that everything is fine. Self-esteem is rooted in being ourselves, even if we suck today.

Being ourselves will help us find supportive relationships. Possibly some romance. I say romance because it is possible to have consenting sex and still be a duplicitous jerk. This is what I call shit-mouth. If we've got shit coming out of our mouth that we know is manipulative, mean, deceptive, or intentionally ignorant, then we've got shit-mouth. While engaging in shit-mouth banter, there is no fucking way we're gonna make real friends or get laid more than once per vagina. Our semi-erect wieners might wibble outside of a girl's wet spot, but she ain't gonna call us back.

Shit-mouth sets a standard for how much of an asshole we are. To reduce shit-mouth, try only medium sized boundary intrusions, and stop with the racist jokes. If you're pushing a 6 to 10 on the shit-mouth scale, rein it in before accidentally instigating violence. There ain't a quality woman alive happy to have sex with a scrappy cocky dick-faced prick who chirps like an angry rooster. That is not self-esteem; that is being a scary little dick that ain't got any pussy to cry on. Men can't just take out their anger on any person who looks at them sideways. Find healthy outlets, dude.

Step 1: Go fuck yourself. How much masturbation is too much? It doesn't matter. You are always there for you, you know? Isn't that special? Doesn't that fill you with a warm feeling of consistent love? You and your special little guy, all cuddled in bed, watching lube trickle down the ass cheeks of your favorite porn star. Yes. Go fuck yourself. Twice daily. This is the only justifiable number that allows for maximum masturbation and minimal shame when she asks awkwardly, "How many times a day do you masturbate?" Twice. Make it a fact.

Step 2: Try dating, then stop. Most of us are big softies who keep trying to date. Get a thick skin to rejection. Despite almost certain rejection, keep going out and meeting people in a safe, consensual fashion. Unless you are physiologically screwed up, internet dating is awesome! Go become better at writing congruent sentences; take a writing class to improve your dating profiles. There will be women there, and you might get a chance to talk with one. Just know when to stop and move on.

Step 3: Pimp yourself online. Lazy, arrogant, and underemployed aren't especially marketable characteristics. Too bad, hey? However every negative virtue has an antithesis. If you are lazy, write it as patient. Arrogance can mean courageous. Underemployed can mean you are an excellent cook and fisherman. Embrace your negative traits to counterbalance them consciously. You aren't lying, you're just treating yourself more kindly.

Step 4: Arrest cardiac disease. Heart attacks aren't sexy. If your lifestyle has led to cholesterol buildup, have personal health discussions with your partners before risking procreation. A sickly lion is never the first pick of the pride, so get healthy. Get your health together brother; your health is a number one priority for relationship maintenance.

Society foolishly validates hyper-sexuality in males, but this myth has led us to isolation, competitiveness, and prioritizing sex over our total health. We believe in flawed male behavioural protocols so sincerely that our group-status is elevated by our capacity for recklessness and stupidity. This is unfortunate because men have much more to offer than just their balls and dumb stunts. Our circumstances might be regrettable, but it doesn't mean we can't change. Self-esteem comes from many sources—sex is just one.

Did you even know that?

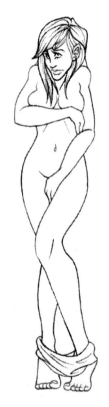

28.
Getting Nakey
101

Ah yes, this part. Positive self-regard will be important when getting naked with company. We get naked alone every day before we masturbate and before we shower. We see our bodies in the mirror all the time. Yup. Men naked. We don't need to think about it generally, but we need to practice thinking about ourselves naked if we want to get proficient with sexy company.

The base line I work with is that more or less, after four drinks men are fully capable of stripping down without a second thought. We tend not to think about men naked because in movies and porn naked men are a subject of comedy or disembodiment. Being naked in reality is a whole different thing. So let's do it with a little more pizazz. This doesn't mean go streaking. It means being comfortable naked, sober, and with some character.

Intimacy is the part before and after sex. A good connection can get a pair so damn aroused that pants are just too confining. When genitals start to do their thing, eventually complete nudity will be achieved. At that point, not a lot of viewing of bodies takes place. It's mostly just mouths, faces, and inches of skin. Once we are thoroughly participating in sex, our self-image becomes less important than our libido. As our sex life with a partner progresses in familiarity, more viewing takes place. That is when body image and the flaws we try to hide might begin to surface.

Fucking in long-term relationships requires a lot of being seen naked. Nudity will lead to intimacy through the inherent feeling of vulnerability in nakedness. Men cannot separate sex from emotion otherwise there would never be batterers. The more sex that we have with one person, the more we become an emotionally bonded creature. Unfortunately, this can be dangerous in a macho male peer group (aka: pussy whipped). Once we are comfortable with our nakedness, we will be better prepared to have healthy relationships. This is because, in sex, we submit our body and ego to the judgement of a lover. They will find our inadequacies, thus we are encouraged to continue to improve. Let's get comfortable in our bodies so that we can get comfortable with our flaws. Our bodies are the most obvious place to start self-improvement. Our relationship to our body is more critical than our body itself. How we treat our bodies is a reflection of how we feel about ourselves. Subsequently, how we feel about ourselves reflects on how we view others.

Do you dance? Are you comfortable being seen as a little bit goofy and sensitive? Do you tense up when you pass strangers in the street? Are you an emotional eater? Do you get self-conscious? Can you comfortably articulate your flaws? Do you have intrusive thoughts that prevent you from sustaining an erection? These are all signs that you might have hang-ups around getting naked.

When we just fuck, we intentionally skip the soul-penetrating intimacy stuff. Getting naked is easy when it's wrapped up into spontaneous passion off the moment; however that shit fades when we start getting into long term relationships. I advise caution and honest communication when in the reckless pursuit of achieving multiple sex partners at once. Firstly, having multiple relationships is stressful because we are taking on the emotional needs of many people. Secondly, it sets a man up for lot of interpersonal conflicts. Regardless in the sexual moment, let's be just as gung-ho about the relationship (in whatever context) as we are about the sex. That puts a man on track to better naked sessions.

Problems arise in nudity when we feel unattractive, disrespected, or insecure. This is a long-developed mental trap. Recovery will take some time. Confidence comes when we realize we can pick ourselves back up. Consider going to the Pride parades to witness the vast capacity for bodily expression. This helps us free ourselves from our body image hang-ups. By accepting our body type, we give a boost to our confidence. There are so many body types, and to not have them all represented is a shame. We are so oversaturated by pornography that it has made us more self-conscious rather than self-accepting.

Use light humor to expose and dispel difficult emotions that arise from nudity. When that once fabulous sex life seems to dry up, remember that there is some comedy in male nudity. Work some funny stuff into a later-stage relationship sex routine. If that is a dance routine, a puppet show, chocolate panties, or a few jokes, do it. Anything that makes a little laugh and hug happen will put us closer to that warm, juicy, tenderness we're seeking. Don't ever whine about no sex; earn it and talk about it with your partner. Seek to understand why sex is not happening and work on it. Obvious sex-inhibitors include addiction, numbness, hygiene, non-communication, over-working, and anger.

There could be some deep personal stuff that's making intimacy and nakedness difficult for you. This is unfortunate if you are not seeking help. Identifying hang-ups is an important step. Recovering from relationship loss or other kinds of trauma takes significant effort and by doing so, you will free up energy to redirect onto more important personal functions.

So here, have a few tips about getting naked.

Step 1: Pick a theme song. This is your official "I was transformed into a woman for a day and spent the night down at the docks picking up sailors" disco strip song. Practice it when no one is watching. Learn the beat changes, and rehearse a dance routine in living room. Add a lip-sync portion and plan a couple moves, then bam, you're golden. This will give you access to some comedic sexuality that can aid in your sex practice. When the time comes to dish out this private dance, laughter will be guaranteed, and her adoration may follow.

Step 2: Respect your physical form. While you are looking at her going "Mhmm yum," she might be doing the same to you, so really, who is sexy? The answer is that you both are. I know, right? Weird, the sexual equation actually includes you. The male form counts. Yup, you have underutilized your 45% stake in global sex appeal (LGBTQ folks pick up the 10%). Sadly the hyper-vigilant focus on the female body has left the male body looking like passed over cattle. I dare you to be sexy to the greatest possible extent without bravado.

Step 3: Fact and performance. Dick size and physique are facts and will be relayed in gossip. Whatever. The date will also be relayed in gossip, so make them positive and memorable. Sexual performance is also valid gossip. All that is deemed "good" is the origin of repeat sexual encounters. Sex quality will be understated and referrals don't exist. The best sex is too good to share. By being comfortable with your body and familiar with your best strokes, you will increase the likelihood of repeat performances. On the flip side, horrible sex or sexual violence is impossible to overlook.

Step 4: Less is more. The number of sexual partners you have will be a function of perceived capacity for loyalty. Likewise, a hundred strokes-per-minute does not guarantee good sex. Good sex comes from harmonizing, detecting subtleties, and confident physical prowess. Sexy masculinity should be understated but confidant. Give lots of high quality attention to the right person, not shitty attention to lots of people. By being endearing, understanding, supportive, and perceptive, we get better at getting naked with others.

Detecting subtleties is a key to quality sexual relationships.

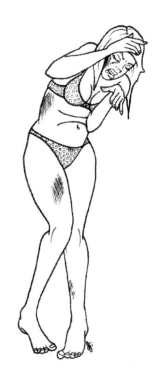

29.
Desperately in Love;
That Bitch!

Men have got it bad when they starting raging at a woman he's apparently in love with. It's so damn ironic it pains me. It kills partners. And it terrorizes the domestic sphere. What do men not understand? Violence is for the military, not an intimate relationship. Violence is not simple to recover from. Fact. Women have legitimate safety boundaries. That invisible line is crossed the moment we raise our voices.

When you are no longer getting what you want from a relationship, instead of blaming your lover, find a new strategy. After she's dumped you come up with a plan and don't fly off the handle. Don't ever bank on reconciliation after a rage—it's pathetic. If your lover wants to get the fuck away from you, the relationship ain't gonna work out, ever. Strategize a recovery, fool. Don't spend any time calling that woman a C-U-Next-Tuesday. Yes, you were hurt, rejected, and sad because of the relationship fell apart. Don't compound the problem by saying ignorant bullshit like this:

"Fuck that bitch. If she'd only listen to me, she would take me back." She did listen, but you speak like a self-righteous idiot when you are suppressing emotional bullshit. That bullshit spewing out your mouth is toxic. When you are firing emotional bullets and yelling to drown-out your spouse's unpleasant revelations, you are totally fucked up. Exit before you escalate.

"I hate her for making me feel this way." The only one you can control is yourself. Your actions have impacted your spouse and she has responded by leaving. She is not obliged to continue a relationship with an emotionally immature man who fails to take responsibility for himself. There were probably many opportunities to modify your behaviour and change. Now that you've been dumped you are angry at yourself for not taking action earlier. So you think you are stupid, but you are not. You're only stupid if you get violent. Maybe the breakup was inevitable. Maybe the flaws were critical to your understanding and she gave up trying to push against them.

"I'm going to win her back," means you probably are sickened by the thought of her fucking someone else. Enter creepy stalking behaviour and rebound perversion. It is hypocritical of a man to respond to divorce with a ferocious eagerness to fuck and not extend that same courtesy to the ex. There are many men who are excellent at helping to rehabilitate woman's sexual intrigue after a shit-head boyfriend gets dumped. Stereotypically, men may move faster in having sex again after a relationship, but she will recover emotionally more quickly and therefore will have better sex sooner. Yes, her sex is going to be better than yours, and there ain't anything you can do about it. Sure, you can get hotheaded and creepy and do something stupid. Ha! But you can't win her back.

When we find that we are simultaneously angry and in love with a woman, we are a danger to ourselves and others. Our behaviour could be augmented by our intake of substances and that can really throw a man out of whack. Watch out for being mean to close friends and expect inexplicable drops in energy. If we give in to blunt, meaningless rage, we'll find ourselves on the receiving end of punishment and nowhere closer to a solution. Revenge is not a healthy way to finish a relationship. Leave that to lawyers if necessary.

If you find yourself feeling angry and in love, be very careful with how you spend your days. These conflicting feelings arise when an important relationship falls to shit. Identifying that these very strong, conflicting feelings exist will help you to not screw yourself up worse.

> Step 1: Avoid compounding problems. Keep it together when shit hits the fan. You can be pissed off, sad, upset, and disappointed but if you go berserk and fuck more shit up, you'll just suffer more. When it gets bad, let that rage out in a fashion that doesn't incur personal liability, violence, or police intervention. Try fishing or hitting the gym, community groups, or emergency meditation.

> Step 2: Mood swings. "You'll be fine" is bullshit. When you say that, you repress what's actually happening. What happens when you take these emotional short cuts is that you never get comfortable in the middle. You become either emotionally "fine" or "pissed," nothing in between. In fact, life has a lot more to offer than these emotional poles. There is a fucking rainbow of emotions involved in a divorce. When middle or transitional emotions go unrecognized (such as grief), we are left with only the extremes.

> Step 3: Letting go. Losing love is similar to experiencing a death. It is possible to cohabitate in the same city as someone you've been in love with. If you don't feel that way, that is problematic. There is no good way to let go of someone you love, but it has to be done: research grief. Be as graceful as possible, because a traumatic break-up becomes baggage in future relationships.

Step 4: Reflect. There was probably a lot of unrecognized conflict in your past relationships. Before running into your next dysfunctional relationship, take a couple weeks or months to learn from what the fuck happened. Once the emotions die down, the personal journey will become apparent in hindsight. Be able to articulate in calm words how your last relationship broke down and what you learned from it. Your next girlfriend will appreciate it.

Just chill. Love visits all men at some point, but it might fade away without care. Relationships must be treated as fragile. Once it's gone, it's gone—like dust in the wind. New loves exists, but fix some of your shit before you dive right in there again.

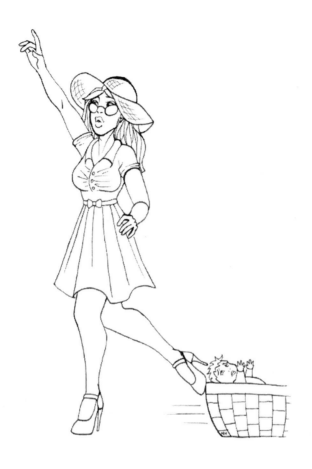

30.

The Run Away Dad (or Absent Father)

Man alive! You came first, buddy. That little human creature, which will erupt from her vagina nine months post-fucking, is a little version of you. Maybe you forgot, or didn't realize in the moment, that the act of ejaculating into a human female will result in a wee little baby being born. A precious, delicate, and a real-life embodiment of you. Yikes. You? Yes, really.

Now, we can't reverse time and abortions (though rightfully available) are not a super-happy choice to have to make. Considering we (hopefully) enjoyed the sex, an abortion is real downer. Going to an abortion clinic after a great summer romance is similar to coming home from Lollapalooza to find our father dead from alcohol poisoning. So, when the conversation arises about unplanned pregnancies, pause, listen, don't freak out, and phone your dad—if he's available. He'll have some ideas about how not to fuck it up. In the case of no-dad, go ahead and visit a local clinic. Ask questions about what the fuck you're supposed to do. I'd hope they'd refer you to some counselling or at least a pamphlet.

Let's play pretend and say that we didn't sincerely adore this mother-of-your-child. Oh boy, so basically we're inextricably linked to a woman who we don't really like, indefinitely. She may turn out to be a real C-U- Next Tuesday. Obviously, we aren't going to get much sympathy from the community if we fuck off after impregnating a local uggo. Clearly we were screwing around, man. Leave the lady-uggos for gentle-uggos.

Don't just fuck incidentally. Fucking uggos and having one-night stands isn't a path to transcendent sex-magic. That's called emotional bingeing; nobody in these relationships benefits long-term. It becomes tragic when two irresponsible people accidentally become parents. Though I hear ugly skips a generation, stupidity does not. The difference between me fucking uggos and the average dick is that I have an annual condom budget, get explicit consent, have sex sober, and develop a positive relationship culture *before* fucking. Douche bags, wear those little rubber things on your goddamned infectious impregnating tool! Come out the gate seeking supportive and kind lovers; be prepared to give back in kind.

Babies: accidents happen but they can also be planned for. However we impregnate, it will be followed by an unprecedented emotional rollercoaster called Fatherhood. There is a whole field of medicine dedicated to the obstetrics (that's lady-baby science) but few give a shit about the male process of birthing a child—for obvious reasons.

Men just get fat and emotional during pregnancy. It's what happened to my brother and my buddy Dave. Both of them still don't shave often enough. Men will probably also become doubtful of themselves and afraid they'll never see another man-camp again. Men might feel the loss of his bromances. Relish these fleeting moment of being not-a-father. They will be gone soon, and will never, ever return.

By becoming a father, men are trading their rampant and misguided self-gratification for the immortalization of their genetics. Breeding might give a man an actual (biological) purpose in life! It's not a bad deal, but men will be somewhat fearful of babies for sure. Over and above the crushing fear of inadequacy, he'll dread the loss of his youthful freedom. All of his imaginary fears are still very real. But once the face of his wee (potentially ugly) little baby converts him into a dad, his fears become visceral and real. Fatherhood will hit men on the head like a backpack of Barbies (aka: a steep learning curve). Bewildering moral conflicts will suddenly surface in our man brains: mortality, continuity, responsibility, dedication, loyalty, consistency, discipline, tolerance, temperance, patience, and respect for stuffed animals. Sorry dude, but that's just the start of a sexually successful fatherhood.

For fathers who want their sons to succeed, macho masculinity has no place in domestic care—it hurts everyone. Fathers-of-sons, do not replicate your boys into stupider versions of yourself. Our grandfathers' values were extremely prejudicial, violent in their ignorance, and toxic for men's health. We must let that generational stupidity go. Let it go! Bring on the next generation of thoughtful males by being fathers who recognize the inherent emotional isolation of pattern male behaviour. Dangerous stunts, drinking and driving, excessive sexuality, objectification of women, and rash violence serve no purpose to a full-grown man. Raising boys macho will not result in well-liked boys. Do not let our boys become jerks by not being jerks ourselves. Boys are culturally sexualized very early. The results of premature sexual development are gruesome. If our boys are learning that happiness comes from inside a girl and not from inside himself, then we are raising emotionally dependant fools—(in other words, your kid is an idiot). Happiness doesn't come out of vaginas, fatherhood does.

We must take excellent care of ourselves in order to show to women that we can take excellent care of our children. If we skip self-care, then our boy will not learn how to take care of himself, either. Healthy parents make healthy children—even if they are uggos.

Just don't freak out. Though we are not prepared right now, we will be. When a man is put under pressure, he tends to perform out of fear of emasculation. The alternative is crumpling, which is not very manly. If a man runs from his duty of raising a child, he is not a healthy man and should consider counselling. A man who fails to rear his child presents a biological profile of a beta-male who simply lucked out on the genetic continuity lottery. Unenlightened betas aren't worthy of copulation; however, they do manage to fuck sometimes. This is how it came to be known as "getting lucky". Running away from a major responsibility like fatherhood is an inexcusable gap in masculine integrity. Alpha-males will be able to sniff out this cowardice, females will be subconsciously repulsed, and the beta will solidify his feelings of inadequacy.

Even if we strongly dislike the woman who birthed our child, keep relationships civil, functional, and even kind. Conflict resolution does not necessitate a romantic reunion, but it will help minimize toxic emotions like bitterness and hate. This is important because anger towards the ex, begets resentment towards the child. Don't make it worse by becoming abusive. We must take care of ourselves and let her take care of herself independently. Let the child into your heart, soul, and wallet.

> Step 1: Abstain from fucking women you don't like. Wow! Whoa. What? You can't have a pornographic sex life without incredible communication skills. Therefore, lots of talk will be needed to get to the sex we imagine. For a less tortuous experience, actually enjoy the company of the women you are seeking to fuck. Despite what the movies tell you, men don't fuck nearly as much as you'd think. Decode the messages about masculine norms and make your own choices. Men are not supposed to fuck all the time; that would be catastrophic. Rampant male sex is a myth. Casanovas are rare and very subtle. Most men have far less sex than you'd think. Slow down your pursuit and add a little class. You watch too much porn. Sexual relationships develop over time with trust, communication, and effort.

> Step 2: Less is more. A hundred sexual partners isn't a very cool thing to mention to a date. You might be in sexual competition with your bro but women won't think that's attractive. Having had a few relationships and a couple of flings will come off as more

endearing than a long list of fuck stories. Also, having a terabyte wank-bank won't ever impress anyone.

Step 3: Condoms or fatherhood. Wear condoms, you disgusting jackass. Work condoms into your sexy moves. Get it out early so that she can relax knowing it's there. The alternative of condoms is possibly herpes or fatherhood. Being reliant on a woman taking birth control is like hoping the pilot took her anti-psychotics. We only find out she's skipped her meds after the fuck-up happens. Take pregnancy into your own hands by wrapping a rubber around your wiener.

Step 4: Being a dad. As a non-parent, parenthood looks busy, expensive, and super annoying. I wager there are some pretty profound benefits, especially once you are old-as-fuck. Regardless of the togetherness factor, when you have children, uphold a supportive relationship with the other parent. Child-rearing makes up for our general lack of purpose otherwise. Therefore, you need that child just slightly less than it needs you. Becoming a father is a part of the cycle of masculine validation. Not only does your child prove that you have a penis, it also proves that you are willing to buffer some unpleasantness for the sake of someone else. It is very virtuous. No big deal.

In closing, be responsible before responsibility is forced upon you. It will be less uncomfortable that way.

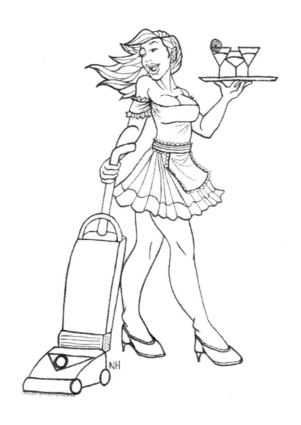

31.
Good House-Husband:
Refine Your Skills and Attract
Your Dream Woman!

Hygiene is frequently over-looked as fundamentally appealing. It seems obvious now because you've read it, but actually try to apply that information to your real life. This includes flossing your fucking teeth as well as cleaning your kitchen and washing your sheets. Dick.

Get those dishes done, clean your supply underwear before you run out, and always remember to feed yourself. Granted, a spotless home and an immaculate wardrobe aren't exactly possible every day, but effort is still required. There are a lot of slobby people out there, but that doesn't automatically validate every-one living like shit. Imagine that you meet a woman and move in together. Your state of filth will present fodder for a regular argument and be grounds for many sexless nights. Whose responsibility is it to clean up our mess? As a lifetime bachelor (or soon to be), this answer is obviously: you.

Rather than get upset with your own lethargy, just man up and do the fucking chores. It's good co-habitation practice. Home maintenance is a guaran-teed life problem. This includes dusting, toilet bowls, clean sheets, and stubborn shower residue. That's on top of the handyman shit involving power tools. If you are not doing these typical chores to a respectable level, your home will not be attractive. Your friends and lovers will need a high tolerance for garbage when-ever they come over. Unfortunately, our homes are a reflection of ourselves, so everyone who comes over will know you're a gross slob. What do you do then? Never see anyone?

It is in our filthy homes that we hope to do most of our fucking and long-term relationship development. Therefore, instead of frantically scrubbing the shit stains off the porcelain throne while Windexing toothpaste out of the sink at zero-hour; actually develop higher standards of domestic hygiene. Schedule deep cleaning weekly.

Once you've settled into a long-term live-in relationship you will probably be inclined to leave your underpants lying around and get lazy. Stop. Don't. Be mindful of the impact on that has on a relationship. Becoming not disgusting will be a difficult transition for the average bachelor. Your ugly habits (such as undisposed-of cum-filled tissues) will become quickly magnified when you are under regular spousal supervision. This could be a good thing! When a person consistently witnesses your dumbass behaviour, they might inadvertently curb your stupidity. This is probably what most men are hoping for. This is a very divorceable mental trap. Somehow we will succeed to get a woman into our lives and she'll unconsciously facilitate our remedial evolution (at her own expense).

145

It happens all the time. What is much more interesting, however, is how a man will fuck up a good thing by taking it for granted and be left with nothing.

Ah, well. Statistically speaking, we need not worry about our first wife's mother. So in between that first failed relationship and our next one, refine that glorious domestic talent. Make lasagna! Invest in some shoe polish! Visit the local garbage and recycling receptacle. Clean tricky spaces that require moving your furniture and action figurines. And of course, clean the bed sheets. They are covered in ass, wiener, flesh, sweat, drool, semen, public hair, and snack residue.

The most difficult part of any household to maintain is the kitchen. Frankly, it has the most moving parts and opportunities for congealed goo. I advise men to begin there. The dishcloth is a long and trusted tool (it too requires regular laundering). There is no technical learning curve to master, nor any specialty education required to regularly employ a dishcloth. Neither are there significant financial barriers to the benefits of the dishcloth. The broad applications for the device in question are virtually limitless. Other factors, such as absorption, solvent distribution, texture, size, and quality, make the dishcloth an extraordinary household tool. Take hold of that age-old domestic godsend, the mighty dish cloth, and clean up your filthy castle.

Here are some places you should keep clean and a few strategies to getting there:

Step 1: Get the gross spots. There are obvious gross spots you should know about but probably don't. With a little ingenuity, you'll be able to find them. The real challenge is controlling the natural smell of your home. This is a combination of many things such as air flow, B.O., festering urine, or soggy rotten Cheetos behind the microwave. Take action if you happen to notice a distinct fragrance of beef emanating from your oven. Also, take action when black speckles turn up on the yellowed panels in the recesses of your refrigerator. Shoes are also smelly so do something about that, like build a wooden bin and paint it. (The sawdust and paint will work in your favor as you craft a new home aroma)

Step 2: Cooking and dishes. To encourage some financial prudence, I suggest you take up dining at home. All those cooking shows do is make you want to go spend a lot of money at that fancy-pants famous chef's restaurant. From a financial and a nutritional standpoint, this is not sustainable for you or a family. Be prepared to cook, not just occasionally, but every single day forever. Follow that up with some light kitchen cleaning and you are on track to being useful.

Step 3: Fruits and vegetables. Nothing says success like a bowl full of fruit! Nothing makes happy bowel movements like a crisper full of vegetables. Fruit is nature's candy, and vegetables its doctor. Put effort into eating colourful plates (make veggie-rainbows, you lazy motherfuckers), but if that fails, make shakes.

Step 4: Coupons and unexpected expenditures. A sausage might cost you a dollar, and two sausages might cost you a dollar somewhere else. Follow the grocery flyers and subscribe to coupon services everywhere. Plan to save money. Expect unexpected expenses. Differentiate between needs and wants. Always track your expenses, read your bills, and find out methods to avail cash for what matters.

You can, in fact, have an important role in the economics of your household. Even just beginning to think that way will set you apart from the average dude. Only the best men will find the best women. Therefore, to achieve your delusions of grandeur, you must become an excellent house-husband, lover, and home economist to get your dream woman.

The men falling short of this will find themselves equally paired, or not paired at all. If you are a fool dreaming of "marrying-up" (as they said in bygone days), then you had better get back to the kitchen and roast up a turkey.

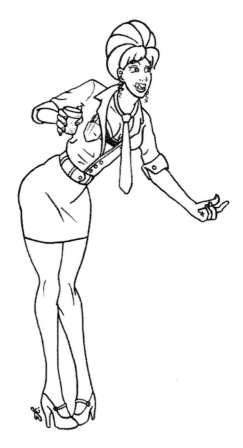

32.

The Workplace
Sex Snafu

Well, well, well. I can't say that I've ever been the perpetrator of a workplace sex snafu. However, I have been on the receiving end one. It had the effect of creating a very tense work environment.

Sexual harassment ruins good working relationships. Once upon a time when I was working in a café, there was this flirtatious under-aged woman who would purr at me, invite me out, and ask to come over. She would squeeze her shoulders, smack her ass, bat her eyes, and say some pretty scandalous stuff. Man alive! It was tense. I'd show up to work hyper-vigilant, and very nervous. My boss and co-workers laughed at this predicament, so I quit.

If a man is unfortunately inclined to date a co-worker, he only gets one chance to ask her out. After one rejection, it's done. I don't believe there is anything wrong with respectfully asking a co-worker on a date, but we've got to be clear with our intention and accept that one rejection equals an unlimited number of them. I have a general philosophy: avoid dating co-workers all together. It is lazy. Moreover, it's potentially boring as fuck in deeper conversations. Inevitably our sex-life will be penetrated by our work-life, and that is fucking preposterous. Just don't. Dating co-workers says to everyone around that we didn't actually try to develop an independent community removed from our employment.

Women add immense value to our workforce. By sexualizing co-workers, it is not the co-workers' productivity that suffers, it is yours. You are the one distracted and daydreaming. You are the one who will lose your job. You are the one that will have to explain your reason for leaving your job to your next employer. Having a work-life balance becomes tricky when our sex life reminds us of work.

So, eyes up, ears open, silence that sexist mouth, and date elsewhere. Do not interrupt women when they speak. Simply by virtue of her newness to a once male-dominated industry, her input will be vastly more original than yours. Your loud talk and tedious defensiveness show an obvious attempt to uphold a masculine environment and satisfy men's insecurity with change. Just fucking relax! Eventually it will happen, we'll have female bosses. There is no need to talk smack about female competition in the workplace—it will distract you from success. Work frats will just drive each other crazy trying to figure out how to outmaneuver hardworking women. (Pro tip: work with them.)

Men can ruin everything by being creepy at work and online. There are many industries where leering, pervy men lurk inside gross corporate cultures—not just heavy industry. Industries such as finance, technology, military, construction, and law enforcement have long histories of being male-dominated. This is beginning to change but men's resistance produces tragic levels of chauvinism and unnecessary conflict. If we are working in an industry where sexism exists, we work in an environment where we are unlikely to find supportive friends. When we see that our buddies are rude to women or they yammer on about their cock's priorities, assume these guys are toxic to our hope of dating and workplace happiness. Crossing the line of sexual harassment is easy when our peer groups are filled with dumb fucks. But we really confirm our dependence on prostitution when our first impulse around women is to glad-hand their asses and vocalize about our sexual impulses. The more we sexually harass women, the further we get from being around them.

When seducing, be like a lithe and gentle sex tiger. Though this could include showing up with marinated beef, what I mean is, imagine that you are a worthy and exquisite creature. Like a tiger. Romance is not dead. Women just have more choices now (so do we) and aren't required by God to tolerate men's bullshit. Respond to these new mating challenges by actually evolving rather than being an insecure prick. In this era of women's emancipation, men must become responsive in a positive fashion. Anything to the contrary and a man will find himself disappointed with the outcome of his sex life. Women will leave us, women will sue us, women will slander our reputation, and women will reject us. This is the same power men have had over men forever. Men's self-esteem is inextricably linked to his ability to have women in his life. So why be such a fucking douche bag to women? Is it because males are super dependent on women for their emotional-sexual satisfaction and biological continuance? Do men resort to sexual aggressiveness to hide failures and increase their odds of (manipulative) sex?

If you and your guy friends agree that it is totally reasonable to act above the reproach of women, you are stupid, wrong, privileged, and dangerous. Get this right or expect to live alone.

Step 1: Aggression never works. There is absolutely no guarantee that you will find what you seek. It is frustrating. It is upsetting. It is a lonely and depressing thought. The solution for this loveless condition falls to your effort and ability to create supportive friendships. Using aggression to pursue or maintain a love interest is a dead-end.

Step 2: Pressured sex is rape. Give up after the first rejection. No means no, and anything less than "Oh my god yes, I want you right now" is insufficient. Being rejected or being denied sex is absolutely normal. If you find that you react with anger or violence to sexual rejection, you are banned from dating until you've got your emotions under control.

Step 3: Cease verbal objectification. Lusty homosocial sex talk about women does nothing for a dude's ability to be accepted by women. Homosocial sex-talk only serves to a build a misogynistic pact between us and our friends. Toxic dudes will hold onto that pact, whereas the best dudes will find girlfriends and move on. A healthy dude's monogamy will inhibit him from being friends with old toxic buddies. When a guy moves on from his old friends they will call him pussy-whipped. Fuck those dudes! They are lonely, angry, jealous, desperate, and hopeless. A healthy romantic relationship will provide far more support, far more encouragement, and far more sex—unless we're fucking our buddies.

Step 4: The predatory female. If you are an excellent man, women will respond. The ideal man's seduction is virtually invisible. He withholds his touch until the long-anticipated moment of first contact. This is very sexy. Seduction occurs through the nose (literally olfactory & pheromones) and we subconsciously detect those we are attracted to. It cannot be forced. If you are fit, well fed, and intriguing, women will be interested in meeting you. Even more so, by being accommodating in your philosophy, kind in your social confidence, and clear in your goals, you will attract the right kind of women. Pursue your life, be open to women, and possess complex subjects in your mind. Women are around. Examine your social magnetism. When flirting, less is more; smile and be thoughtful. When that long-anticipated moment of first contact arises, that is when you act. She will have been watching you for quite some time.

The hunting tiger-man lays and waits patiently. He is prepared knowing that his skills are sharp and his choice mate is nearby. He is alert and carefully positioned. There is only this one chance. It's hot and he must conserve his energy. He carefully calculates his approach. The prospective mate will either run or embrace him. There is only one way to find out: he cautiously approaches his target.

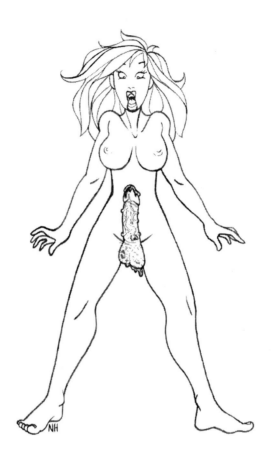

33.
The Infected Penis

Somehow it happened: we got a wart on our dick. Or maybe it's an in-grown hair, or burning piss, or jock itch, or yeasty excretions—the point is we don't know if we don't get tested. There is a long list of symptoms attributed to potential sexual ailments, and my favorite is the mythical and figurative dick-leprosy.

We can't conceal this problem to lovers and still be considered a responsible adult. Yes, it's a major self-esteem hit to be diagnosed with herpes. However, the self-esteem hit quadruples when we infect other people. Men are impregnators and carriers. By not getting tested for sexually transmitted infections, our dick-psyche can become toxic and dangerous. Not only might we ignorantly transmit a permanent infection to our lover, we might impregnate a person too. Great, now we've infected not one, but two life forms with our toxic cock. Congratulations, we've officially made the world a worse place and entangled someone else in our shitty healthcare maintenance.

It is staggering how few men get tested. It's laughable insecurity really, but it's too gross to actually be funny. What are we so afraid of? Are we afraid of a little prick, or of the test results? Either way, we are all fucking idiots for not taking care of ourselves. We can't act like an ostrich when we start having dick-related healthcare problems.

There are many ways to enjoy dick-leprosy. It can come from an immovable and deep-seated emasculation, or from a feeling of sexual isolation and a lifetime of stagnation. A physician can help with all sorts of dick leprosy except the ones we ignore. If men are totally fortified in their fearful ignorance, I recommend they permanently commit to celibacy or counselling. When we ignore glaring medical problems and do not seek help, we become dependent on women to persuade us to go. With high divorce rates and rising intolerance for brutish male behaviour, men will probably be on their own while they self-destruct. At that point, I sincerely hope their buddies come through for them.

Buddies: help your buddies. Do so freely. Real friends help each other, including getting them in for STI testing. We don't have to tell our guy friends about our herpes (unless we're fucking them) but it's time for men to go do health prevention stuff in groups.

Know thy penis well. Asking why and how our sex life impacts our well-being is a worthwhile exploration. Frivolous sex makes men a walking infection risk if they are not tested. Too much of a good thing makes it less special, Mr. Big Dick. Why women like crude and scary dudes is beyond my comprehension— I'd guess that woman can manipulate bravado and wield it like personal power, but I don't know. Never the less, is men's rampant pursuit of sexual validation really benefiting him in the long run? Isn't it more like the communication of a lonely boy who wants a personal connection so badly that he'll hurt other people to get it? Men need boundaries and values attached to sex or they'll fail to recognize that relationships require respect and dignity.

Okay, whether you've got a problem with your dick or not: get tested. An infection is obviously upsetting but pretending it doesn't exist will make it worse. The inevitable outcome of dick-leprosy will occur—permanent emasculation. By not maintaining a healthy cock, the opportunities for you to use it will rapidly decrease.

Here's a few ways to curb dick leprosy:

Step 1: Get tested. Oh God, yuck, gross. Get tested, like, today. Do it now.

Step 2: Dick-brain relationship. Men benefit from having access to two brains. That's why we are so damn ingenious. Unfortunately, we only have enough blood to operate one at a time. Let your condoms and consent be taken care of cognitively long before your dick-brain takes over. If you jump into sexy time and neglect important safety measures (like condoms, tests, and consent), you'll suffer some severe consequences. Examine your dick-brain relationship and teach it to articulate itself before it becomes overthrown with short-sighted passion.

Step 3: Sad days infected. If you have outbreaks on your dick, go show a doctor. There is a lot to learn from doctors when it comes to dicks and the emotions associated with dicklessness. Speaking to a doctor will give you less of a downward mystery spiral and more of an optional ladder to recovery.

Step 4: Saying uncomfortable words. The opposite of honest disclosure is an emotionally retched, spiritually damning, and genuinely guilty experience. Silence is the worst thing you can do when it comes to concealing dick-related health problems from lovers. Prudence is a virtue (though it is a tricky word) in man-terms. It means: stop, think, think, act, and be responsible. The words you are hesitant to say must be said. Speak the truth and let the cookie crumble. That moment of discomfort is far less shitty than a lifetime of knowing you've infected someone else.

Get tested. Tell your friends you went! Don't share your results. Lie by omission in public but be honest with your lovers. If you have never been tested, that is ridiculous and gross—everyone agrees. Try to be less fucked. Don't get all gloomy and angry; just go manage the problem of not knowing.

Get tested! For fuck sakes.

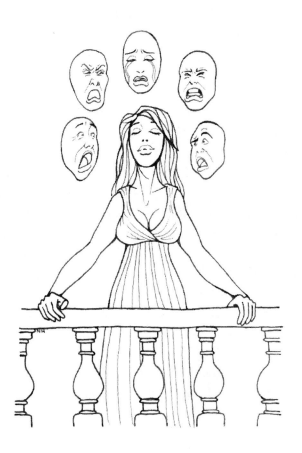

34.

Hormones,
The Hourly Man Cycle

Women's hormonal cycle is monthly (like the moon), but men's hormonal cycle is daily (like the sun). For example men bear the common cold with so much needy want of comforts that even his dogs grow weary of his whining. When men are ill, distressed, or distracted, they will behave sporadically because of these hourly hormonal spikes. Likewise, for no evident reason, sometimes men can flip their lids in a situation where at other times they have reacted calmly.

Flash testosterone quickly exhausts itself. Men tend to recover, apologize, and move on without a second thought. Through self-reflection they can begin to learn the shadow side of this behaviour and learn to choose helpful responses rather than hormonal reactions. As they become informed, they will discover that there is emotional pretense to all of their actions. If a man can recognize that he is exploding on a regular basis, he may be able to pause and prevent his emotional blowout by accepting his hourly hormonal man-cycle.

It is good for a man to get fired up once a day, every day. We have a daily motivating impulse (aka: a morning woody) to do, to make, and to act. It can be extremely helpful. But where does the productivity go? Probably a tissue. For the most part, youthful males are blessed with an erection every day. Every day men's bodies have literally got something to do, but masturbation fatigue can kill our motivation. Masturbation should not be removed from the daily calendar but should be limited to once in the morning and once in the evening so that ejaculation fatigue is easy to recover from. Clearly our desire to shoot sperm is a hormonal impulse so go ahead and masturbate, but recognize that there is still a lot to do every day.

Our regular morning erection is a call-to-action, but it is age-sensitive. This is called the Chronic Erection Period (CEP) when our man-hormones spike daily. How we take care of our physical and mental health determines the length of time we get to enjoy regular boners and daily hormonal inspiration.

During CEP, men will feel elevated levels of virility, enthusiasm, and hope. Ah, hope. It is so easy to have during CEP, but it fades. It fades ever so subtly until we die. This is why men with CEP act so dynamic (or hormonal and emotional). When hormonal spikes are present, a man's amazing dick-brain is vacillating between two objectives—sex and doing stuff. The sexual brain seeks orgasms but the non-sexual brain seeks satisfaction through many complex objectives. Ejaculations, however, are not the deepest motivations of man, not by a long shot. His non-sexual brain is far more dominant than we are told to believe. A man is foolish to channel all his energy into sex during CEP because he denies the complexity of his maturing goals.

Men's daily emotional irregularities may be related to CEP or lack thereof. When men experience emotional spikes (in behaviour) it can range from binge eating to yelling. These urges need to have productive outlets because otherwise they'll just find victims—sometimes it's ourselves. Men subconsciously understand other men's dormant emotional volatility, so we naturally avoid provoking each other (even if it means offering help). Men interact with little or no emotional input in order to avoid triggering hormonal spikes. It is uncomfortable for men to be around emotional men because we have poor emotional intelligence. This has been reinforced by how men love to appear emotionally stable, even if they're not. The result has been the self-stigmatization of the emotional male experience, which is the root men's behavioural volatility. Ostensibly, male hormone spikes can come at any time during the day and are provoked by our balls and channeled by our complex objectives.

Every day men have emotional spikes, especially during CEP. But men like being ultra-hormonal (so much, even if it's gone) that they have replaced passion with recklessness and motivation with numbness within the cult of masculinity—just to keep up appearances. It is a troubling delusion, because that passionate-motivated masculine impulse has been drastically oversimplified. What was once represented by families, hard work, community effort, and togetherness has been overcome by a pornographic urge to ejaculate all the time. An over-simplified dick impulse invalidates a man's holistic experience, hurts other people, and offends the man himself for thinking so lowly of his life. How can we channel this energy into something helpful or productive? Start with the self.

I recommend self-satisfying labours, volunteerism, any physical exertion, or active relaxation.

Men are sexual all the time, but in most circumstances that is irrelevant. Use the power of CEP that comes every morning, and immerse yourself in a personal objective. That is how to channel CEP and how to respond appropriately when hormones aren't required. It is catastrophic for relationships when we let our daily hormonal cycle become bravado. Hormones dwindle but reputation remains. If a man has a high number of sexual impulses daily, I suggest he create a long list of activities. Unless we are inclined to become known as perverted goons, I suggest men develop a respect for their hormonal cycle.

Use that hormonal influence to your advantage. Do not use it to intimidate people. Flaunting testosterone is for wrestlers and douche bags earning their donkey punch in prison. Enjoy creating a master plan for your dick-brain; yet know that happiness exists in the present moment too. Work your man-magic to achieve that which you seek through daily effort.

Step 1: Don't say that shit. We get all excited and say (or tweet) shit we didn't think through—it can be rude, racist, sexist, or disgustingly out-of-place. It was a bad choice, and we recognize that, and we are sorry. However, gentlemen, what we fail to learn is that sometimes this kind of outspokenness can be of immense benefit when channeled correctly. This comes in the form of advocacy and intervening as a bystander. Our words can have a profoundly positive impact on our lives. So yes, speak out, but speak thoughtfully because words can hurt people.

Step 2: Watch that reflex. An emotionally charged, snap response can land us in a lot of shit. If we are getting amped up, jacked up, or hot headed, ask for a moment to cool down. Enter a breathing exercise. Just that one pause or little bit of humble explanation is sometimes enough to stop a situation from escalating.

Step 3: Dick Dick Dick Dick Dick! Men have far less sex than one might think. Man's priorities are diverse and complex. Seeking satisfaction is a fair argument when it comes to motivating a man to move mountains. However, in relationships there are far fewer mountains than interpersonal conflicts. Sex might not rain abundantly on our cocks—think that one through for a while. However, if and when we are in a relationship, what will happen is that we begin to rely less on our sex-brain and start exercising our complex-objectives brain. It takes finesse to learn about intimacy. By neglecting intimacy (in practice), we'll never learn how to sustain a long-term sexual relationship—because sex is never the primary purpose of a long relationship. The purpose of togetherness is to validate our complex needs. If we over-simplify our hormonal impulse and neglect to channel it into anything productive then we're fucking ourselves over.

Step 4: Old creepy men. I don't know what to expect in retirement, but I have met a ton of old people. It would appear the impulse remains long after the hormones are gone. Creepy old men like to flirt and feel connected to women. Though his capacity to fuck has radically diminished, the elderly male still loves female company. So, in the long run, men desire women's company much more than for just their sex. If we neglect our complex needs today, we'll be cursed to remain sexless, ugly, and alone—this is the difference between cute old man and creepy old man.

In conclusion, human males might very well die drunk, sad, and isolated if they don't become aware of their complex needs and how behaviors impact health. This is a fate worth fighting against. Let's reinvent the socially acceptable stupidity of men. We want to draw in good friends and kind partners by starting with ourselves. Just as we are, just as they are, we must go forth and do what we do best in relationships. If you seek a sexy and happy existence, listen to yourself and let romance and manliness become close friends. Be more of what your body is asking from you. What do you want? How are you going to get there? Is it honestly working?

Every day you are changing, and every erection presents an unlimited number of possibilities.

Good Luck with the Dick

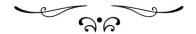

You read a book! Well done. I will send you a fucking certificate—maybe (there'd have to be a quiz). What now? You've probably forgotten most of it, so you can re-read it with a highlighter or you can re-gift it to a friend or (if you're female or gay) give it to an ex as a divorce gift. Shit, you've already bought and read it, I'm totally fucking satisfied. I guess it would be nice to hear what you thought. So do that. I want to improve and learn more about this kinda stuff, so ya, be in touch—internets and whatnot. There is a relationship model in the back pages, try filling that out, if and when you ever get a love life.

It is worth talking about sex, health, and masculinity. The best thing you can do now is chat it up. Get real with your mental and physical health; start with friends. Find a lifestyle that you can be proud of, or just something that works for you as you are right now.

Masculinity is evolving. Though I have my doubts (especially about myself), I wish you luck and hope that you will be successful in adapting quickly enough to pass on your wisdom. The odds have just increased slightly. Sex, happiness, and life-long supportive relationships are hard-earned. This demands thoughtful contemplation; otherwise you can pretty much anticipate struggling with the fear of dying drunk, and alone forever.

Introduction to the Levis-Pimm Relationship Model

The writing down of information should go back and forth. Both participants must take each step. As a relationship evolves what was written will change. Re-do it again in a few weeks, then months, then years. Reveal only what you are comfortable revealing at this time in your relationship. Skip step 21 & 22 in non-sexual relationships*. Apply caution, as this model isn't tested by any fancy school or university. It was developed privately to resolve the fallout of a workplace romance; Levis and Pimm are ordinary citizens, not doctors or counsellors.

Step One – establish a supportive relationship.

Step Two – introduce LP Relationship Model to partner as an optional communication tool.

Step Three – upon agreement get different coloured pens and a copy of the diagram.

Step Four – put your names in your respective circles.

Step Five – write something you **value** about your partner (underneath your partner's name).

Step Six – write an **activity** that you know your partner loves to do (on their activities line).

Step Seven – write something you **value** about yourself (beside your name).

Step Eight – write an **activity** that you love you do (on your activities line).

Step Nine – pause for conversation. Fill in the blank after "**we want:**" together.

Step Ten – write down a **challenge** that you will face during this relationship (on your line).

Step Eleven – write down what you are **offering** to support this relationship (on your lines).

Step Twelves – write down **expectations** of yourself (on your side of the Venn diagram).

Step Thirteen – write down **expectations** of your partner (on their side of the Venn diagram).

Step Fourteen – Discuss mutual **expectations** and **joint needs**, write them in the middle.

Step Fifteen – write what you are **seeking** within the context of the relationship (bottom corners).

Step Sixteen – address **fears** by writing down your worries and uncertainties (top corners).

Step Seventeen – Add to mutual **challenges** and mutual **activities** together (on the middle lines).

Step Eighteen – review, add, clarify, and discuss.

Step Nineteen – revisit in a week, resolve red flags, opportunities, and partner-pleasing.

Step Twenty* – write down a few kinks or sex fantasies (under the scale on your side)

Step Twenty-one* – Fill in weighted sexual preference percentage M/F (ie: 50/50 = bisexual).

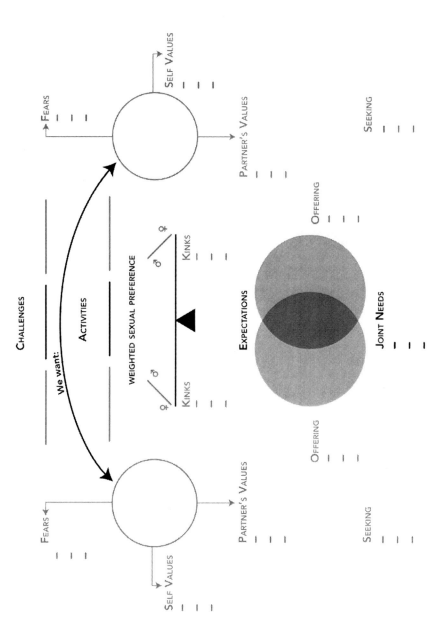

The Levis-Pimm Relationship Model©

CPSIA information can be obtained at www.ICGtesting.com
Printed in the USA
LVOW11s0452051115

461153LV00002B/43/P